Disclaimer Notice:

Please note the information contained within this document is for educational and entertainment purposes only. All effort has been executed to present accurate, up to date, reliable, complete information. No warranties of any kind are declared or implied. Readers acknowledge that the author is not engaged in the rendering of legal, financial, medical, or professional advice. The content within this book has been derived from various sources. Please consult a licensed professional before attempting any techniques outlined in this book.

By reading this document, the reader agrees that under no circumstances is the author responsible for any losses, direct or indirect, that are incurred as a result of the use of the information contained within this document, including, but not limited to, errors, omissions, or inaccuracies.

CONTENTS

Introduction

According to the World Health Organization (WHO), 1.9 billion adults worldwide over the age of 18 years are overweight.

Obesity can be a serious health problem as it can cause type-2 diabetes, heart disease, musculoskeletal disorders like osteoarthritis, and even some types of cancer. It can also cause gallbladder disease, high blood pressure, gout, and sleep apnea. Worldwide, obesity is getting worse. WHO estimates that it has almost tripled since 1975.

Sleeve gastrectomy, first performed in 1990, is a very effective treatment for obesity. It is a surgical process recommended to those with a BMI (Body Mass Index) of 40 or higher. People with a BMI of 35-39.9 can also go for the gastric sleeve surgery if they have a serious weight-related health issue.

Thank you for downloading this book.

Here, I will discuss gastric sleeve surgery in detail to prepare you for the process.

<u>This Is What You Will Find In This Book</u>...

- Detailed understanding of sleeve gastrectomy
- Preparing for the surgery
- Foods and medications that are allowed and disallowed
- A detailed guide on the various stages of recovery
- Possible weight loss indicators from the surgery

Finally, I will also share many mouth-watering gastric sleeve recipes that are all easy to prepare. For each recipe, I will provide a list of ingredients and detailed step-by-step instructions.

I am sure you will find this book very useful. Happy reading!

Chapter 1 – What is Sleeve Gastrectomy?

Sleeve gastrectomy, which is also known as Vertical Sleeve Gastrectomy or Bariatric Surgery, is a weight-loss surgical procedure. The surgeon will insert small instruments through laparoscopy into your upper abdomen. There will be many small incisions. Parts of the stomach will be removed in the process. Surgical staples will be used to join together the remaining parts of the stomach.

The process creates a 'sleeve', which gives the surgery its name. The new stomach is much smaller in size, about the tenth of the original.

Sleeve Gastrectomy is recommended to obese people who must lose weight urgently. It is recommended to those who are facing obesity-related health problems like high blood pressure, diabetes and sleep apnea. It is also suggested to people who have high cholesterol, heart disease, are suffering from infertility, or the gastroesophageal reflux disease. The process reduces the risk of all these conditions substantially.

It is an option for people who cannot lose weight in any other way or keep gaining back the lost weight. Sleeve gastrectomy is like the last resort for these people.

Qualifying for the Surgery

Ideally, those with a BMI or Body Mass Index of 40 or higher may think of going for this surgery. A 40 plus BMI is considered to be extreme obesity. Those with a BMI between 35 and 39.9 can also consider sleeve gastrectomy, especially if they have a serious weight-related health issue. In some instances, the surgery may also be considered with a BMI between 30 and 34 if the weight-related health problems are very serious in nature.

Sleeve gastrectomy is less invasive compared to gastric bypass surgery because the intestinal tract doesn't have to be reconstructed here. It is simpler and safer.

It is usually a safe procedure. There can however be some fluid leakage from the stomach and bleeding. But they are temporary and can be fixed easily.

The death rate with this surgery is less than 0.1%, which is lower than a hip replacement surgery or gallbladder operation.

The gastric sleeve surgery has become very popular worldwide in recent years. It is particularly popular with severely obese people with weight-related health issues. The process is a good option for those who cannot lose weight in any other way or when they manage to shed the excess pounds but it keeps coming back.

Surgery can be an efficient way to lose excess weight, but it is also necessary to commit to a healthier lifestyle after the procedure. It is particularly important to pick the right foods after the process.

Chapter 2 – Preparing for the Gastric Sleeve Surgery

The surgery is carried out in a hospital. You may have to stay there for 1 or 2 nights.

If you qualify, the healthcare team will provide instructions to prepare you for the surgery. Lab exams and tests might be recommended before the process.

Food, Medications

Supply the doctor a list of all vitamins, minerals, medicines, and dietary or herbal supplements you may be taking. Eating and drinking restrictions may be imposed. There can also be restrictions on some medications. For instance, always mention if you are taking blood-thinning medications because they can affect bleeding and clotting. The medical team may change the routine for these drugs.

If you are suffering from diabetes, talk with the doctor who is managing your medicines and insulin. The professional may make adjustments or offer specific instructions.

There are some other precautions to take.

1.   Stop smoking at least 12 weeks before the surgery. You may be given a nicotine test if you use tobacco.

2.   Start exercising as soon as you plan the process. A physical activity program will help you during the surgery and will also improve your health.

3.   It is also good to plan the recovery, even before the surgery. Get help at home. Those who opt for the surgery usually miss work for about 4 weeks.

Before and During the Surgery

You have to change into a gown before entering the operating room. Inside, you will be anesthetized before the surgery. This will keep you asleep during the surgery.

How the surgery is conducted depends on the doctor's or the hospital's practices and also on individual health conditions. Usually, it is performed laparoscopically (key-hole). Small instruments are inserted through different small incisions in your upper abdomen. However, in some instances, open incisions may also have to be made.

The surgery may take up to 2 hours. You will then be transferred to a recovery room where the medical staff will monitor your condition.

Most people start walking just 3-4 hours after the surgery.

After the Surgery

During release from the hospital, the medical team will make many diet change recommendations that must be closely followed. You will also be told to take a vitamin B-12 injection, calcium supplement, and multivitamin.

Frequent medical checkups will be carried out to monitor your health, especially in the first 3-4 months after the surgery. This includes bloodwork and lab tests.

There can also be some changes in your body in the first 6 months. Your skin can become excessively dry, you may feel tired, there can be body aches, and you may even see some hair loss. Some people also report frequent mood changes. All this happens because your body is still adjusting with the rapid weight loss.

Chapter 3 – Gastric Sleeve Recovery Guide

The medical team will issue instructions to prevent complications before you leave the hospital. This includes specific instructions on when you can resume regular activities. Every person recovers differently, but usually, it takes a few weeks before you can go back to work. Remember to stay properly hydrated. Vigorous physical activities should be avoided completely for the first 4 to 6 weeks.

The First Week After Surgery

The pain, if any, will be very mild. Simple pain medicines can solve the issue. Most gastric sleeve patients experience pain during the first week. It gradually subsides after this. Inform your surgeon if you have pain even after the first week.

Avoid physical activities. Do not climb stairs or lift anything. However, you can start driving after the first 7 days.

You may feel exhausted. Don't worry because this is mostly due to the restricted diet immediately after the surgery.

3 Weeks After the Surgery

Most gastric sleeve surgery patients can return to work after 3 weeks. But don't exert yourself too much because your body is still recovering. You won't have any noticeable pain. There can, however, be an itchy or tugging feeling.

You may be allowed light workout activities. This could be daily walk for 5 to 10 minutes. However, there will be strict restrictions on any type of weight lifting.

1 Month After the Surgery

There shouldn't be any complications at this time. By this time, you will feel much lighter. There will be a noticeable difference. There shouldn't be any pain, which means, you will need fewer medicines.

The doctor will allow you to take some solid foods. But there will still be many dietary restrictions.

3 Months After the Surgery

You can now start doing activities like swimming, yoga, and dancing because the wounds have healed and your body has adjusted itself. Prescription medications may also be completely stopped. However, the doctor may still recommend some supplements and vitamins.

Modest physical activities will also be allowed. But only 20 to 30 minutes a day. You may start lifting light weights as well. Some people report hair loss at this time. Don't worry. This will stop soon.

6 Months After the Surgery

By the end of the sixth month, you would lose most of the excess weight, which will make you look a lot thinner.

You are ready to start a rigorous and high-paced workout regime. You can visit the gym and do almost everything. In fact, it is best that you exercise for 4-5 days a week. Cycle, walk briskly, run, or swim if you cannot go to the gym.

1 Year After the Surgery

Severely obese people will lose 70 to 90 pounds by the end of the first year. This, of course, depends on the pre-surgery weight.

There shouldn't be any problems at this time. Make sure to continue eating healthy foods. Junk and greasy foods can cause health problems.

Chapter 4 – Sleeve Gastrectomy Diet

Those who opt for the surgery must follow a special diet both before and after the process. The pre-surgery eating plan must start 2 weeks before the scheduled date.

This will be a strict diet where the focus will be on consuming fewer carbohydrates from potatoes, pasta, and sweets. You will mostly have to take vegetables, lean proteins, and low or no-calorie fluids. In many cases, a daily calorie goal is set.

Two days before the surgery, you must switch to a liquid diet. You may have no-sugar protein shakes, decaffeinated tea or coffee, water, broth, and sugar-free popsicles. Avoid carbonated or caffeinated beverages. Remember the following –

- No high-sugar beverages like sodas and juice
- Reduced intake of saturated fats
- Restricted intake of high-carb foods like pasta, desserts, bread, and potatoes
- No binge eating, smoking, and drinking alcoholic beverages
- Exercise portion control
- Protein powder and protein shakes are allowed
- Take a multivitamin daily

After the Surgery

Immediately after the surgery, you will be put on soft and smooth foods. Solid intake will come with time. Here is a table that explains this very nicely.

However, the schedule will vary from one person to another. Some people will always progress faster than others.

Time	Regimen	Best Foods
24–48 hours	Only fluids at room temperature	Half-cup servings of liquid. This is gradually increased to 8 cups a day
3–7 days	Liquid foods are introduced	Soy drinks, milk, unsweetened yogurt
1–2 weeks	Mashed or pureed foods	Mashed fish, soups, low-fat cheese, pureed vegetables and fruits, thin cereals like oats, skim milk
2 weeks	Soft foods can be introduced	Scrambled or boiled eggs, soft meatballs, peeled and soft fruits, peeled and cooked vegetables
1 month	Solid foods	Fresh vegetables and fruits, legumes, whole grains, bread
2 months	Resume balanced, regular diet	Soy products, high protein foods, lentils, eggs, meat, vegetables and fruits, hard cheese, protein supplements

Chapter 5 – Foods to Avoid

There are some foods that will increase the risk of complications after gastric sleeve surgery. So they should always be avoided. Stay away from the following –

- Dry and hard foods that will be difficult to swallow after the surgery
- High glycemic index foods like potatoes, rice, and bread that can increase the blood sugar level
- Calorie dense beverages and foods like cakes, ice cream, milkshake, and chocolates
- Sugar-sweetened and carbonated drinks like soda
- Chewing gum and foods that cause flatulence like beans

Tips and Guidelines

Remember the following for quick recovery.

1. Eat more frequently but small amounts of food every time
2. Eat and chew slowly
3. Stay away from concentrated sugars
4. Avoid non-nutrient calories
5. Avoid processed, fast, and fried foods
6. Stay away from alcohol
7. Use a food processor or blender to puree food
8. Differentiate between appetite (emotional) and hunger (physical)
9. Stay properly hydrated
10. Take multi-vitamin and B complex
11. Avoid nonsteroidal anti-inflammatory drugs like aspirin, ibuprofen, and naproxen
12. Start walking, swimming, and dancing after the doctor recommends

Chapter 6 – How Much Weight Can You Lose?

Most people can shed between 60% and 70% of their excess body fat. It comes back a bit because the sleeve will expand slightly after the surgery. But over the long-term, they can still reduce around 50% of the extra body weight.

The weight is lost in two ways. You will eat less because the size of the stomach is now smaller and it can only hold a limited quantity of food. You will feel full more quickly. The process also removes the stomach's part that produces a hormone that increases appetite. This reduces hunger pangs.

The weight loss is usually the maximum in the first few months. But you will keep losing weight until the end of the first year. Some people keep losing even beyond this, making them appear their leanest by the end of the second year.

- **First 2 weeks** – 10 to 20 pounds of excess weight. On average it is about 1 pound a day.
- **First 3 months** – 35% to 45% of the excess weight.
- **First 6 months** – 50% to 60% of the excess weight.
- **The first year** – 60% to 70% of the excess weight by the end of the first year.

Breakfast Recipes

Guava Smoothie

Servings: 2
Cooking Time: 5-7 Minutes
Ingredients:
- 1 cup guava, seeds removed, chopped
- 1 cup baby spinach, finely chopped
- 1 banana, peeled and sliced
- 1 tsp fresh ginger, grated½ medium-sized mango, peeled and chopped
- 2 cups water

Directions:
1. Peel the guava and cut in half. Scoop out the seeds and wash it. Cut into small pieces and set aside.
2. Rinse the baby spinach thoroughly under cold running water. Drain well and torn into small pieces. Set aside.Peel the banana and chop into small chunks. Set aside.
3. Peel the mango and cut into small pieces. Set aside.
4. Now, combine guava, baby spinach, banana, ginger, and mango in a juicer and process until well combined. Gradually add water and blend until all combined and creamy.
5. Transfer to a serving glass and refrigerate for 20 minutes before serving.Enjoy!
Nutrition:Per Serving: Net carbs 39.1 g;Fiber 7.8 g;Fats 1.4 g;Fatsr 2 g;Calories 1

Breakfast Kale Muffins

Servings: 8
Cooking Time: 30 Minutes
Ingredients:
- 6 eggs, lightly beaten
- 1/2 cup unsweetened coconut milk
- 1/4 cup chives, chopped
- 1 cup kale, chopped
- Pepper
- Salt

Directions:
1. Preheat the oven to 350 F/ 0 C.
2. Spray a muffin tray with cooking spray and set aside.
3. Add all ingredients into the mixing bowl and whisk to combine.
4. Pour mixture into the prepared muffin tray and bake for 30 minutes.
5. Serve and enjoy.
Nutrition:Per Servings: Calories 95 Fat 7 g Carbohydrates 2 g Sugar 1 g Protein 5 g Cholesterol 140 mg

Avocado Cherry Smoothie

Servings: 3
Cooking Time:20 Minutes
Ingredients:
- ½ ripe avocado, chopped
- 1 cup fresh cherries

- 1 cup coconut water, sugar-free
- 1 whole lime

Directions:
1. Peel the avocado and cut in half. Remove the pit and chop into bite-sized pieces. Reserve the rest in the refrigerator. Set aside.
2. Rinse the cherries under cold running water using a large colander. Cut each in half and remove the pits. Set aside.
3. Peel the lime and cut in half. Set aside.
4. Now, combine avocado, cherries, coconut water, and lime in a blender. Pulse to combine and transfer to a serving glass.
5. Add few ice cubes and refrigerate for 10 minutes before serving.
Nutrition value per serving: Calories: 128, Protein: 1.7g, Total Carbs: 17g, Dietary Fibers: 3.8g, Total Fat: 8g

Low Carb Cottage Cheese Pancakes

Servings:1
Cooking Time: 5 Minutes
Ingredients:
- ½ - cup low-fat cottage cheese
- ¼ - cup oats
- ⅓ - cup egg whites (2 egg whites)
- 1 - tsp. Vanilla extract
- 1 - tbsp. Stevia in the raw

Directions:
1. Pour curds and egg whites into the blender first, at that point include oats, vanilla concentrate, and a little stevia.
2. Mix to a smooth consistency.
3. Put a container with a bit of cooking shower on medium warmth and fry every hotcake until brilliant on the two sides.
4. Present with berries, without sugar jam or nutty spread.
Nutrition: Calories 20fat 1.5g;carbs 19g;sugar 5.5g;protein 24.5g

Sweet Millet Congee

Servings: 4
Cooking Time: 1 Hour 15 Minutes
Ingredients:
- 1 c. Millet
- 5 c. Water
- 1 c. Diced sweet potato
- 1 tsp. Cinnamon
- 2 tbsps. Stevia
- 1 diced apple
- ¼ c. Honey

Directions:
1. In a deep pot, add stevia, sweet potato, cinnamon, water and millet, then stir to combine.
2. Bring to boil over high heat, then reduce to a simmer on low for an hour or until water is fully absorbed and millet is cooked.
3. Stir in remaining ingredients and serve.

Nutrition: Calories: 136, Fat: 1g, Carbs: 28.5g, Protein: 3.1g

Vanilla Egg Custard

Servings: 6
Cooking Time: 30 Minutes
Ingredients:
- 4 large eggs
- 2 tsp vanilla extract
- 2/3 cup splenda
- 12 oz can evaporated milk
- 1 cup milk
- ½ cup Nutmeg, grated

Directions:
1. Preheat the oven at 325 F.
2. Place six ramekins in baking tray and set aside.
3. Add vanilla, splenda, eggs, evaporated milk and milk in blender and blend until smooth.
4. Pour mixture into the ramekins then pour enough water in baking tray and bake in preheated oven for 30 minutes.
5. Serve chilled and enjoy.

Nutrition:Per Servings: Calories: 255, Fat: 8.4 g, Carbohydrates: 29.5 g, Sugar: 29.5 g, Protein: 9.4 g, Cholesterol: 144 mg

Strawberry & Mushroom Sandwich

Servings: 4
Cooking Time: 10 Minutes
Ingredients:
- 8 oz. Cream cheese
- 1 tbsp. Honey
- 1 tbsp. grated Lemon zest
- 4 sliced Portobello Mushrooms
- 2 cup sliced Strawberries

Directions:
1. Add honey, lemon zest and cheese to a food processor, and process until fully incorporated.
2. Use cheese mixture to spread on mushrooms as you would butter.
3. Top with strawberries. Enjoy!

Nutrition:Per Servings: Calories: 180, Fat: 16g, Carbs: 6g, Protein: 2g

Mushroom Frittata

Servings: 2
Cooking Time: 30 Minutes
Ingredients:
- 6 eggs, lightly beaten
- 2 oz butter
- 2 oz green onion, chopped
- 3 oz fresh spinach
- 5 oz mushrooms, sliced
- 4 oz feta cheese, crumbled
- Pepper
- Salt

Directions:
1. Preheat the oven to 350 F/ 0 C.
2. Whisk eggs, cheese, pepper, and salt in a bowl.
3. Melt butter in a pan over medium heat.
4. Add mushrooms and green onion to the pan and sauté for 5-10 minutes.
5. Add spinach and sauté for 2 minutes.
6. Pour egg mixture to the pan.
7. Bake in preheated oven for 20 minutes.
8. Serve and enjoy.

Nutrition:Per Servings: Calories 680 Fat 56.7 g Carbohydrates 8.3 g Sugar 4.3 g Protein 38 g Cholesterol 612 mg

Avocado Shrimp Salad

Servings: 4
Cooking Time: 15 Minutes
Ingredients:
- 1 ripe avocado
- 1 tbsp Tabasco
- 1 tsp ranch dressing
- ½ cup yogurt
- 1 lb shrimp, cooked
- 1 grapefruit, cut into sections

Directions:
1. Combine together Tabasco, ranch dressing and yogurt.
2. Place shrimp, avocado and grapefruit in large bowl.
3. Pour dressing over shrimp and avocado mixture.
4. Serve and enjoy.

Nutrition:Per Servings: Calories: 226, Fat: 10.2 g, Carbohydrates: 11.2 g, Sugar: 4.7 g, Protein: 24.2 g, Cholesterol: 164 mg

Farmer's Egg Casserole With Broccoli, Mushroom, And Onions

Servings:12
Cooking Time: 40 Minutes
Ingredients:
- Nonstick cooking spray
- 2 teaspoons extra-virgin olive oil
- 1 onion, diced
- ½ cup chopped mushrooms
- 2 cups roughly chopped broccoli florets
- 12 eggs
- 2 tablespoons low-fat milk
- ½ teaspoon dried oregano
- ½ teaspoon dried basil
- ¼ teaspoon dried thyme
- 1 cup chopped or shredded cooked poultry breast, such as leftover turkey or chicken, canned chicken breast, or turkey lunch meat (nitrate-free)
- 1 cup shredded Swiss cheese
- ¼ cup shredded Parmigiano-Reggiano cheese
- Post-Op
- 1 (3-by-4-inch) piece

Directions:
1. Preheat the oven to 350°F. Spray a 9-by-13-inch baking dish with the cooking spray.
2. In a large skillet over medium heat, add the olive oil. When the oil is hot, add the onion and sauté for 1 to 2 minutes, or until tender. Add the mushrooms and cook for an additional 2 to 3 minutes, or until tender.
3. In a steamer or microwave-safe bowl, place the broccoli florets and 2 tablespoons water. Cover and microwave/steam for about 4 minutes or just until tender. Drain off any liquid and set aside.
4. In a large bowl, whisk together the eggs, milk, oregano, basil, and thyme.
5. Add the cooked vegetables, poultry, and Swiss cheese to the egg mixture and stir to combine.
6. Pour the mixture into the baking dish and sprinkle the Parmigiano-Reggiano cheese over the top.
7. Bake for 35 to 40 minutes, or until lightly browned. Let the casserole rest for 5 minutes before serving.
8. Store leftovers in the refrigerator for up to 1 week. Reheat before eating.
Nutrition: Per Serving (1 [3-by-4-inch] piece): Calories: 147; Total fat: 10g; Protein: 12g; Carbs: 2g; Fiber: 1g; Sugar: 0g; Sodium: 1mg

Apple And Goat Cheese Sandwich

Servings: 1
Cooking Time: 5 Minutes
Ingredients:
- 2 - slices 100-percent whole-wheat bread, toasted
- 1 - ounce goat cheese, at room temperature
- 1 - tablespoons natural peanut butter
- ½ - medium apple, cored and thinly sliced, divided

- ¼ - teaspoon cinnamon
Directions:
1. Spread bit of toast with goat cheddar and the other with nutty spread. Make a sandwich with a large portion of the apple cuts sprinkled with cinnamon.
2. Present with residual apple cuts.
Nutrition: Calories 408;fat 17g;carbs49g;sugar 15g;protein 17g

Cherry Avocado Smoothie

Servings: 3
Cooking Time: 5 Minutes
Ingredients:
- ½ ripe avocado, chopped
- 1 cup fresh cherries
- 1 cup coconut water, sugar-free
- 1 whole lime

Directions:
1. Peel the avocado and cut in half. Remove the pit and chop into bite-sized pieces. Reserve the rest in the refrigerator. Set aside.
2. Rinse the cherries under cold running water using a large colander. Cut each in half and remove the pits. Set aside.
3. Peel the lime and cut in half. Set aside.
4. Now, combine avocado, cherries, coconut water, and lime in a blender. Pulse to combine and transfer to a serving glass.
5. Add few ice cubes and refrigerate for 10 minutes before serving.
Nutrition:Per Serving: Net carbs 17 g;Fiber 3.8 g;Fats 8 g;Fatsr 3 g;Calories 128

California Steak Salad With Chimichurri Dressing

Servings: 2
Cooking Time: 20 Minutes
Ingredients:
- 1.25lb. flank steak
- 1 - tablespoon olive oil
- Salt & pepper to season
- 8 oz. Fresh arugula
- 1 - red onion, sliced into 1" rings
- 1lb. - asparagus, trimmed
- 1 - pint of assorted cherry tomatoes, halved
- 1 - avocado, sliced
- Chimichurri dressing:
- 1 - garlic clove
- 1 - cup fresh cilantro
- 2 - tablespoon red wine vinegar
- 1 - tablespoon lime juice
- 3 - tablespoons olive oil
- ¼ - teaspoon smoked paprika
- ½ - teaspoon red pepper flakes
- Salt & pepper to taste

Directions:
1. Preheat barbeque to medium-excessive heat.
2. Season asparagus and onion jewelry with olive oil and salt.
3. Set asparagus and onion earrings at the fish fry. Barbecue the asparagus for 5 minutes. Flame broil the onion rings for 5 minutes on every facet until scorch imprints show up. Take out and mounted a at ease spot.
4. Add 1 tablespoon of olive to flank steak, rub into every element. Season the two aspects with salt and pepper.
5. Spot flank steak at the barbeque. Flame broil every factor for 3 to minutes. Let relaxation for 5 minutes earlier than reducing.
6. While the steak is resting add the accompanying to a chunk sustenance processor: a garlic clove, new cilantro, purple wine vinegar, olive oil, lime juice, smoked paprika, red pepper quantities, salt, and pepper. Mix till clean and resembles a dressing.
7. Collect the serving of blended veggies, embody crisp arugula, flame-broiled red onion cuts, asparagus, cherry tomatoes, cut avocado, and reduce flank steak to a big serving platter. Present with chimichurri dressing as an afterthought! Topping with a lime.
Nutrition: Calories: 452;sugar: 6g;fat: 32g;carbs: 16g;protein: 36g

Blueberry Greek Yogurt Pancakes

Servings: 2
Cooking Time: 25 Minutes
Ingredients:
- 2 - large eggs
- ¾ - cup plain 2-percent-fat Greek yogurt
- 1 ½ - tablespoons honey, divided
- ½ - teaspoon vanilla extract
- ½ - cup whole wheat flour
- 1 - teaspoon baking powder
- 1 - pinch salt
- ¼ - teaspoon cinnamon
- 1 - cup fresh (or frozen, thawed) blueberries
- 2 - tablespoons natural peanut butter, divided

Directions:
1. In a bowl, beat eggs. Blend in yogurt, 2 tbsp nectar, and vanilla. In another bowl, mix together flour, heating powder, salt, and cinnamon. Add dry fixings to wet and blend to join. Blend in 1/2 cup blueberries.
2. In an enormous nonstick skillet covered with a cooking splash over medium-low heat, drop a stacking 1/4 cup hitter for every flapjack. Cook until underside is dark-colored and air pockets structure on top, around 3 minutes. Flip and cook around 3 minutes more. Rehash with the residual player.
3. Top each presenting with 1/2 tbsp nectar, 1 tbsp nutty spread, and 1/4 cup blueberries.
Nutrition: Calories: 6;Carbs: 54g;Sugar: 25g;Protein: 23g

Egg White Oatmeal With Strawberries And Peanut Butter

Servings: 1
Cooking Time: 10 Minutes
Ingredients:
- ½ - cup rolled oats
- ½ - cup unsweetened almond milk
- 6 - large fresh (or frozen, thawed) strawberries, cored and chopped
- 2 - teaspoons honey
- ½ - teaspoon vanilla extract
- 1 - pinch salt
- 1/3 - cup liquid egg whites
- 1 - tablespoon peanut butter

Directions:
1. In a little pot, heat oats, 2 cup almond milk, 1/3 cup water, strawberries, nectar, vanilla, and salt. Heat to the point of boiling, at that point decrease to stew and cook, blending once in a while, until the blend is thick, and oats are full, 5 to 7minutes. Expel from warm.
2. In a bowl, whisk egg whites until somewhat bubbly. Add cooked cereal to egg whites a spoonful at once, rushing between every option, until oats are completely joined.
3. Pour blend once more into the pot and cook over low heat, mixing always, until oats are thick, 2 to inutes. Be mindful so as not to turn the warmth excessively high so eggs don't scramble.
4. Top cereal with nutty spread.

Nutrition: Calories 412;carbs g;sugar 17g;protein 20g

Blackberry Vanilla French Toast

Servings: 2
Cooking Time: 50 Minutes
Ingredients:
- 4 - eggs, beaten
- ½ - teaspoon vanilla extract
- Salt
- 4 - slices whole wheat bread
- 1 - cup fresh blackberries
- 20 - pecan halves, chopped
- 2 - teaspoons maple syrup

Directions:
1. In a shallow dish, mix eggs, vanilla, and a gap of salt altogether. Absorb cuts of bread egg blend, every cut in flip, till all of the egg is retained.
2. In a big, nonstick skillet protected with cooking bathe over medium warm temperature, consist of the two drenched bread cuts and cook dinner until underside is awesome darker around 3 minutes. Flip and prepare dinner until fantastic dark-colored and quite firm, around 3 minutes extra.
3. Rehash with the staying bread cuts and the rest of the egg combination.
4. Top with blackberries, walnuts, and maple syrup.

Nutrition: Calories 434;fat 17g;carbs 49g;sugar 14g;protein 22g

Wisconsin Scrambler With Aged Cheddar Cheese

Servings:6
Cooking Time: 10 Minutes
Ingredients:
- Nonstick cooking spray
- 8 ounces extra-lean turkey sausage (nitrate-free)
- 6 large eggs, beaten
- ¼ cup fat-free milk
- ½ teaspoon onion powder
- ½ teaspoon garlic powder
- 3 ounces extra-sharp Wisconsin Cheddar cheese, shredded
- Post-Op
- ½ cup
- ½ to 1 cup

Directions:
1. Coat a large skillet with the cooking spray and place it over medium-high heat. Add the turkey sausage and brown it, using a wooden spoon to break it into small pieces, until cooked through and no longer pink, about 7 minutes.
2. In a medium bowl, whisk together the eggs and milk. Mix in the onion and garlic powders.
3. Add the eggs to the skillet. Reduce the heat to medium-low and stir gently and constantly with a rubber spatula for 5 minutes, until the eggs are fluffy and cooked through.
4. Top with the cheese and serve.

Nutrition: Per Serving (½ cup): Calories: 169; Total fat: 11g; Protein: 1; Carbs: 2g; Fiber: 0g; Sugar: 1g; Sodium: 413mg

Almond Peanut Butter Oatmeal

Servings: 1
Cooking Time: 5 Minutes
Ingredients:
- 1/2 cup rolled oats
- 1/2 cup unsweetened almond milk
- 1 tbsp peanut butter
- 1 tbsp unsweetened chocolate chips

Directions:
1. Add all ingredients into the glass jar.
2. Cover the jar with a lid and shake well and place it in the refrigerator overnight.
3. Serve and enjoy.

Nutrition:Per Servings: Calories 369 Fat 20.5 g Carbohydrates 35.9 g Sugar 1.9 g Protein 11.9 g Cholesterol 0 mg

Cherry-vanilla Baked Oatmeal

Servings:6
Cooking Time: 45 Minutes
Ingredients:
- Nonstick cooking spray
- 1 cup old-fashioned oats
- ½ teaspoon ground cinnamon
- ¾ teaspoon baking powder
- 1 tablespoon ground flaxseed
- 3 eggs
- 1 cup low-fat milk
- ½ cup low-fat plain Greek yogurt
- 1 teaspoon vanilla extract
- 1 teaspoon liquid stevia (optional; to improve sweetness)
- 1 cup fresh pitted cherries
- 1 apple, peeled, cored and chopped
- Post-Op
- ½ cup baked oatmeal (recipe)

Directions:
1. Preheat the oven to 375°F. Lightly coat an 8-by-8-inch baking dish with the cooking spray.
2. Mix together the oats, cinnamon, baking powder, and flaxseed in a medium bowl. In a separate large bowl, gently whisk the eggs, milk, yogurt, vanilla, and stevia (if using).
3. Add the dry ingredients to the wet and stir to combine. Gently fold in the cherries and apples.
4. Bake for 45 minutes or until the edges start to pull away from the side of the pan and the oatmeal gently bounces back when touched.
5. Divide leftover oatmeal into airtight glass containers. Refrigerate for up to 1 week for quick and easy breakfast, or freeze.

Nutrition: Per Serving (½ cup): Calories: 149; Total fat: 4g; Protein: 8g; Carbs: 21g; Fiber: 4g; Sugar: 9g; Sodium: 71 mg

Strawberry & Mushroom Breakfast Sandwich

Servings: 4
Cooking Time: 10 Minutes
Ingredients:

- 8 oz. Cream cheese
- 1 tbsp. Honey
- 1 tbsp. Grated lemon zest
- 4 sliced portobello mushrooms
- 2 c. Sliced strawberries

Directions:
1. Add honey, lemon zest and cheese to a food processor, and process until fully incorporated.
2. Use cheese mixture to spread on mushrooms as you would butter.
3. Top with strawberries. Enjoy!

Nutrition: Calories: 180, Fat: 16g. Carbs: 6g, Protein: 2g

Mocha Banana Protein Smoothie Bowl

Servings: 1
Cooking Time: 5 Minutes
Ingredients:
- 1 - large frozen banana
- ½ - cup almond breeze chocolate almond milk, plus more if necessary
- 1 - scoop your favorite protein powder
- 1 - packet instant coffee, if desired
- 1 - cup spinach
- A few ices cube
- Toppings:
- Almond butter
- Toasted almonds
- Chia seeds
- Low-fat granola
- Sliced bananas
- Fresh strawberries
- Carob chips
- Unsweetened coconut flakes

Directions:
1. Include all fixings aside from wanted garnishes to a blender and mix until smooth and rich. On the off chance that fundamental, include more almond milk and additionally ice to arrive at the ideal consistency. The smoothie ought to be genuinely thick so you can eat it with a spoon.
2. Fill a bowl and top with wanted garnishes, for example, chia and granola.

Nutrition: Calories: 272Fat: 4g;Carb: 45g;Sugar: 26.6g;Protein: 20g

Avocado Toast With Cottage Cheese & Tomatoes

Servings: 4
Cooking Time: 5 Minutes
Ingredients:
- 8 - slices hearty whole grain bread
- 2 - cups cottage cheese low fat
- 1 - ripe California avocado sliced
- 1 - tomato sliced
- Salt and freshly cracked pepper to taste

Directions:
1. Lay bread cuts out on an enormous cutting board and tops everyone with ¼ cup of curds. Sprinkle with salt and pepper.
2. Top curds with avocado and tomato cut at that point season with another spot of salt and pepper.
3. Cut bread cuts down the middle and serve.

Nutrition: Calories: 0 ; Fat: 11.9g ; Carb: 63.5g; Protein: 25g

Southwestern Scrambled Egg Burritos

Servings: 8
Cooking Time: 10 Minutes
Ingredients:
- 12 eggs
- ¼ cup low-fat milk
- 1 teaspoon extra-virgin olive oil
- ½ onion, chopped
- 1 red bell pepper, diced
- 1 green bell pepper, diced
- 1 (15-ounce) can black beans, drained and rinsed
- 8 (7- to 8-inch) whole-wheat tortillas, such as La Tortilla Factory low-carb tortillas
- 1 cup salsa, for serving
- Post-Op
- Burrito filling (no tortilla)
- ½ to 1 burrito

Directions:
1. In a large bowl, whisk together the eggs and milk. Set aside.
2. In a large skillet over medium-high heat, heat the olive oil and add the onion and bell peppers. Sauté for 2 to 3 minutes, or until tender. Add the beans and stir to combine.
3. Add the egg mixture. Reduce the heat to` medium-low and stir gently and constantly with a rubber spatula for 5 minutes, until the eggs are fluffy and cooked through.
4. Divide the scrambled egg mixture among the tortillas. Fold over the bottom end of the tortilla, fold in the sides, and roll tightly to close.
5. Serve immediately with the salsa, or place each burrito in a zip-top bag and refrigerate for up to 1 week. To eat, reheat each burrito in the microwave for 60 to 90 seconds. These will also keep well in the freezer for up to 1 month.

Nutrition: Per Serving (1 burrito): Calories: 250; Total fat: 10g; Protein: 19g; Carbs: 28g; Fiber: 13g; Sugar: 1g; Sodium: 54g

Scrambled Eggs

Servings: 1
Cooking Time: 5 Minutes
Ingredients:
- 3 eggs, lightly beaten
- 2 tbsp chives, chopped
- ½ cup ricotta
- 1 tbsp butter
- Pepper
- Salt

Directions:
1. Melt butter in a pan over medium heat.
2. In a bowl, whisk together eggs, chives, ricotta, pepper, and salt and pour into the pan.
3. Gently stir egg mixture until eggs are cooked and scrambled, about 5 minutes.
4. Serve and enjoy.

Nutrition: Per Servings: Calories 464 Fat 34.g Carbohydrates 7.7 g Sugar 1.5 g Protein 31.1 g Cholesterol 560 mg

Steel Cut Oat Blueberry Pancakes

Servings: 4
Cooking Time: 20 Minutes
Ingredients:
- 1½ c. Water
- ½ c. Oats
- 1/8 tsp. Salt
- 1 c. Flour
- ½ tsp. Baking powder
- ½ tsp. Baking soda
- 1 egg
- 1 c. Milk
- ½ c. Greek yogurt
- 1 c. Frozen blueberries
- ¾ c. Agave nectar

Directions:
1. Combine oats, salt, and water together in a medium saucepan, stir, and allow to come to a boil over high heat.
2. Set it to low and simmer for 10 mins, or until oats are tender. Set aside.
3. Combine all remaining ingredients, except agave nectar, in a medium bowl, then fold in oats.
4. Preheat griddle and lightly grease. Cook ¼ cup of batter at a time for about 3 minutes per side.
5. Garnish with agave.

Nutrition: Calories: 257, Fat: 7g, Carbs: 4, Protein: 14g

Berry Cheesecake Overnight Oats

Servings: 1
Cooking Time: 5 Minutes
Ingredients:
- ½ - cup fresh (or frozen, thawed) blueberries
- 1 - teaspoon honey
- ½ - teaspoon vanilla extract
- ½ - cup rolled oats
- ½ - cup low-fat cottage cheese
- ½ - cup unsweetened almond milk
- 12 - almonds, chopped

Directions:
1. In a bowl or container, consolidate berries, nectar, and vanilla and squash with a fork. Include oats, curds, and almond milk, and mix to join. (the blend will be thick and might appear to be dry, yet the oats will relax as they sit.)
2. Refrigerate in any event 6hrs.
3. Servings cold, sprinkled with almonds.

Nutrition: Calories: 6;Carbs: 48g;Sugar: 11g;Protein: 24g

Thai Chopped Chicken Salad With Peanut Vinaigrette

Servings: 2
Cooking Time: 0 Minutes
Ingredients:
- Salad:
- 2 - heads romaine lettuce
- 2 - bell peppers, any color, thinly sliced
- 1 - mango, sliced
- 1 - cup shredded carrots
- ½ - cup roasted and unsalted peanuts
- 2 - cups cooked shredded chicken
- Spicy peanut dressing:
- 4 - tbsp thai peanut sauce
- 2 - tbsp olive oil
- 2 - tsp honey
- 2 - tsp rice vinegar
- 2 - tsp lime juice

Directions:
1. Finely hack the lettuce and cut peppers and mango into slight strips. Toss lettuce, peppers, mango, carrots, peanuts, and chicken.
2. Make the dressing by whisking together shelled nut sauce, oil, nectar, vinegar and lime juice. Taste and change in accordance with your inclination, including more nectar on the off chance that you'd like it all the sweeter or lime juice on the off chance that you'd like it progressively tart.
3. Just before serving, add a large portion of the dressing to the plate of mixed greens and hurl well. Servings a plate of mixed greens with staying half of dressing as an afterthought and add to your inclination.

Nutrition: Calories: 351;carbs: 36g;protein: 19g;fat: 18g;sugar: 23g

Watermelon Quinoa Parfait

Servings: 1

Cooking Time: 20 Minutes
Ingredients:
- 1 - cup watermelon, cut into bite-sized pieces
- ½ - cup cooked quinoa
- 1 - tablespoon fresh mint, chopped
- ½ - cup plain 2-percent-fat Greek yogurt
- 20 - almonds, chopped

Directions:
1. In a bowl, mix together watermelon, quinoa, and mint.
2. In a container or bowl, layer watermelon-quinoa blend with yogurt. Top with almonds.

Nutrition: Calories 411;fat 17g;carbs 42g;sugar 17g;protein 25g

Coconut Cranberry Protein Bars

Servings: 1
Cooking Time: 0 Minutes
Ingredients:
- ¼ - cup unsweetened shredded coconut flakes
- ¼ - cup organic dried cranberries
- ¼ - cup almond butter
- 2 - tbsp almond meal
- 2 - tbsp flax meal
- 3 - tbsp coconut oil
- 1 - tbsp raw honey
- 2 - eggs
- 6 - scoops sfh coconut fuel protein
- Dash Himalayan sea salt
- Optional: 1/4 organic dark chocolate chunks/enjoy life's chocolate chips

Directions:
1. Preheat stove to 350
2. Come to all fixings in a bowl and blend until a batter-like consistency
3. Line an 8x8 preparing dish with material paper
4. Take off batter into a level and even square
5. Prepare for 1to 20 minutes or until somewhat solidified
6. Let cool and cut into squares

Nutrition: Calories 214;fat 12.2g;carbs 8.2g;sugars 3.1g;protein 20g

Hearty Slow Cooker Cinnamon Oatmeal

Servings:10
Cooking Time: 7 To 8 Hours
Ingredients:
- 8 cups water
- 2 cups steel-cut oats
- 2 teaspoons ground cinnamon
- 1 teaspoon ground nutmeg
- Add-ins for protein (per individual serving, limit to 1)
- ½ cup low-fat milk (add before serving or while reheating)
- 2 tablespoons unflavored or vanilla protein powder
- 2 tablespoons nonfat powdered milk or egg white powder
- 2 tablespoons powdered peanut butter
- Add-ins for flavor 8+ weeks post-op (per individual serving, limit to 1)
- ½ cup fresh or frozen berries
- ½ apple, pear, peach, or banana, peeled and sliced
- ¼ cup pumpkin puree
- ⅛ cup chopped pecans, walnuts, or almonds
- Post-Op
- ¼ cup
- ½ cup
- up to ¾ cup

Directions:
1. In a slow cooker, combine the water, oats, cinnamon, and nutmeg. Cover and cook on low for 7 to 8 hours.
2. Choose and mix in one each of your favorite protein and flavor add-ins before serving.
Nutrition: Per Serving (¾ cup, no add-ins): Calories: 1; Total fat: 2g; Protein: 6g; Carbs: 23g; Fiber: 4g; Sugar: 0g; Sodium: 0mg

Pumpkin Protein Pancakes

Servings: 2
Cooking Time: 10 Minutes
Ingredients:
- 2 - large eggs
- ¾ - cup plain 2-percent-fat Greek yogurt
- ½ - cup canned pumpkin
- 1 ½ - tablespoons maple syrup, divided
- ½ - teaspoon vanilla extract
- ½ - cup whole wheat flour
- ¼ - cup rolled oats
- 1 - teaspoon baking powder
- 1 - pinch salt
- ¼ - teaspoon pumpkin pie spice
- 20 - pecan halves, chopped

Directions:
1. In a bowl, beat eggs. Blend in yogurt, pumpkin, tbsp maple syrup, and vanilla.
2. In another bowl, blend together flour, oats, preparing powder, salt, and pumpkin pie flavor.

3. Add dry fixings to wet and blend to consolidate.
4. In an enormous nonstick skillet covered with cooking splash over medium-low heat, drop a loading ⅓ cup hitter for every flapjack. Cook until underside is darker and air pockets structure on top, around 3 minutes. Flip and cook around 3minutes more. Rehash with residual hitter.
5. Top with walnut parts and the rest of the maple syrup.
6. Cool extra hotcakes before putting away in an impenetrable holder in the ice chest as long as 3 days or store remaining hitter in a sealed shut compartment in the ice chest as long as 4 days.
Nutrition: Calories: 415;Carbs: 49g;Sugar: 15g;Protein: 22g

Mushroom Strata And Turkey Sausage

Servings: 12
Cooking Time: 60 Minutes
Ingredients:
- 8 oz. cubed ciabatta bread
- 12 oz. chopped turkey sausage
- 2 cups milk
- 4 oz. shredded cheddar
- 3 eggs
- 12 oz. egg substitute
- ½ cup chopped green onion
- 1 cup sliced mushroom
- ½ tsp. paprika
- ½ tsp. pepper
- 2 tbsps. grated parmesan cheese

Directions:
1. Set oven to 400°F. Lay bread cubes flat on a baking tray and set it to toast for about 8 min.
2. Meanwhile, add a skillet over medium heat with sausage and allow to cook while stirring, until fully brown and crumbled.
3. In a bowl, add pepper, parmesan cheese, egg substitute, salt, paprika, eggs, cheddar cheese and milk, then whisk to combine.
4. Add in remaining Ingredients: and toss well to incorporate. Transfer mixture to a large baking dish (preferably a 9x13-inch) then tightly cover and allow to rest in the refrigerator overnight.
5. Set oven to 3°F, remove the cover from casserole dish and set to bake until fully cooked and golden brown.
6. Slice and serve.
Nutrition:Per Servings: Calories: 185 , Fat: 18g , Carbohydrates: 9.2g, Protein: 2.4g

Berry Muesli

Servings: 2
Cooking Time: 6 Hours 10 Minutes
Ingredients:
- 1 cup oats
- 1 cup fruit flavored yogurt
- ½ cup milk
- 1/8 tsp. salt
- ½ cup dried raisins
- ½ cup chopped apple
- ½ cup frozen blueberries
- ¼ cup chopped walnuts

Directions:
1. Combine yogurt, salt and oats together in a medium bowl, mix well, then cover the mixture tightly.
2. Place in the refrigerator to cool for 6 hours.
3. Add raisins, and apples the gently fold.
4. Top with walnuts and serve. Enjoy!

Nutrition:Per Servings: Calories: 198, Carbs: 31.2g, Fat: 4.3g, Protein: 6g

Quinoa Bowls

Servings: 2
Cooking Time: 25 Minutes
Ingredients:
- 1 sliced peach
- 1/3 cup quinoa
- 1 cup low fat milk
- ½ tsp. vanilla extract
- 2 tsps. natural stevia
- 12 raspberries
- 14 blueberries
- 2 tsps. honey

Directions:
1. Add natural stevia, 2/3 cup milk and quinoa to a saucepan, and stir to combine.
2. Over medium high heat, bring to a boil then cover and reduce heat to a low simmer for a further minutes.
3. Grease and preheat grill to medium. Grill peach slices for about a minute per side. Set aside.
4. Heat remaining milk in the microwave and set aside.
5. Split cooked quinoa evenly between 2 serving bowls and top evenly with remaining Ingredients:. Enjoy!

Nutrition:Per Servings: Calories: 180, Fat: 4g, Carbs: 3, Protein: 4.5g

Strawberry Cheesecake Chia Seed Pudding

Servings: 1
Cooking Time: 10 Minutes
Ingredients:
- ¼ - cup cottage cheese
- 1 - tbs Greek yogurt
- 1 - cup chopped strawberries, divided
- ½ - cup almond milk

- 1/8 - tsp vanilla
- 2 - tsp raw sugar
- 2 - tbs chia seeds

Directions:
1. In a blender, join the curds, Greek yogurt, 2 cup strawberries, almond milk, vanilla, and crude sugar and mix, mix, mix until the blend is totally smooth and lovably pink. You may need to scratch down with a spatula once in the middle. Fill a lidded holder and include the chia seeds, mixing admirably. Let sit medium-term (at any rate 24 hours, the more it sets, the thicker it gets!) In the cooler.
2. The following day when you are prepared to eat it, blend it again to appropriate the seeds equitably and present with the staying 1/cup slashed strawberries. Yum

Nutrition: Calories: 24;Total fat: 8g

Andrea's Hangry Eggs With Cauliflower

Servings:2
Cooking Time: 5 Minutes
Ingredients:
- ½ (10-ounce) bag of frozen cauliflower florets
- 4 thin slices (nitrate-free) deli ham
- Nonstick cooking spray
- 2 large eggs
- Post-Op
- ½ recipe

Directions:
1. Place the cauliflower with 2 tablespoons water in a microwave-safe bowl or steamer. Cover and cook on high for 4 minutes, or until tender. During the last 30 seconds, add the ham to thoroughly heat it. Drain off any water after cooking.
2. Coat a small skillet with the cooking spray and place it over medium-high heat. Crack two eggs into a small dish and set aside.
3. When the skillet is hot, carefully add the eggs. Reduce the heat to medium-low. Jiggle the pan slightly and then allow eggs to cook for 2 to 3 minutes, or until the whites turn opaque and the yolk starts to cook but is still soft in the center. If necessary, use a rubber spatula to adjust the egg slightly to prevent it from sticking. Place the cauliflower on a plate and the ham on top of the cauliflower. Add the eggs, allowing the yolk to spill over the entire dish. Eat immediately.

Nutrition: Per Serving (½ recipe): Calories: 109; Total fat: 6g; Protein: 11g; Carbs: ; Fiber: 2g; Sugar: 1g; Sodium: 378mg

Turkey Sausage And Mushroom Strata

Servings: 12
Cooking Time: 1 Hr. 15 Minutes
Ingredients:
- 8 oz. Cubed ciabatta bread
- 12 oz. Chopped turkey sausage
- 2 c. Milk
- 4 oz. Shredded cheddar
- 3 eggs
- 12 oz. Egg substitute
- ½ c. Chopped green onion
- 1 c. Sliced mushroom
- ½ tsp. Paprika
- ½ tsp. Pepper
- 2 tbsps. Grated parmesan cheese

Directions:
1. Set oven to 400 degrees f. Lay bread cubes flat on a baking tray and set it to toast for about 8 min.
2. Meanwhile, add a skillet over medium heat with sausage and allow to cook while stirring, until fully brown and crumbled.
3. In a bowl, add pepper, parmesan cheese, egg substitute, salt, paprika, eggs, cheddar cheese and milk, then whisk to combine.
4. Add in remaining ingredients and toss well to incorporate. Transfer mixture to a large baking dish (preferably a 9xinch) then tightly cover and allow to rest in the refrigerator overnight.
5. Set oven to 3 degrees f, remove the cover from casserole dish and set to bake until fully cooked and golden brown.
6. Slice and serve.

Nutrition: Calories: 185, Fat: 18g, Carbs: 9.2g, Protein: 2.4g

Carrot Cake Oatmeal

Servings: 1
Cooking Time: 50 Minutes
Ingredients:
- ½ - cup unsweetened almond milk
- 1 - small carrot, peeled and finely grated
- 1/3 - cup rolled oats
- 1 -tablespoon raisins
- 1 - teaspoon honey
- ¼ - teaspoon vanilla extract
- 1 - pinch cinnamon
- 1 - pinch salt
- 1 ½ - tablespoons peanut butter
- 1/3 - cup low-fat cottage cheese

Directions:
1. In a bit pot, be part of almond milk, half cup water, carrot, oats, raisins, nectar, vanilla, cinnamon, and salt. Heat to the factor of boiling, at that point, reduce to stew and cook, mixing sporadically, until thick and oats are stout, 5 to 7minutes.
2. Blend inside the nutty unfold and take out from the heat.
3. Top cereal with curds and extra cinnamon.

Nutrition: ;Calories 3;fat 17g;carbs 51g;protein 21g

Pumpkin Muffins With Walnuts And Zucchini

Servings:2
Cooking Time: 25 Minutes
Ingredients:
- Nonstick cooking spray or baking liners
- 2 cups old-fashioned oats
- 1¾ cups whole-wheat pastry flour
- ¼ cup ground flaxseed
- 2 tablespoons baking powder
- 1 teaspoon baking soda
- 1 teaspoon ground cinnamon
- ¼ teaspoon ground nutmeg
- ¼ teaspoon ground ginger
- ¼ teaspoon ground allspice
- 2 cups shredded zucchini
- 1 cup canned pumpkin or fresh pumpkin puree
- 1 cup low-fat milk
- 4 eggs, lightly beaten
- ¼ cup unsweetened applesauce
- 1 teaspoon liquid stevia
- ½ cup chopped walnuts
- Post-Op
- 1 muffin

Directions:
1. Preheat the oven to 375°F. Prepare two muffin tins by coating the cups with the cooking spray, or use baking liners.
2. In large bowl, mix together the oats, flour, flaxseed, baking powder, baking soda, cinnamon, nutmeg, ginger, and allspice.
3. In a separate medium bowl mix together the zucchini, pumpkin, milk, eggs, applesauce, and stevia.
4. Add the wet ingredients to the dry and stir to combine. Gently stir in the walnuts.
5. Fill the cups of the muffin tins about half full with the batter.
6. Bake until the muffins are done, when a toothpick inserted in the center comes out clean, about 25 minutes.
7. Let the muffins cool for 5 minutes before removing them from the tins. Place on a baking rack to finish cooling.
8. Wrap leftover muffins in plastic wrap and freeze. Reheat frozen muffins in the microwave for about 20 seconds.

Nutrition: Per Serving (1 muffin): Calories: 128; Total fat: 5g; Protein: 5g; Carbs: 18g; Fiber: 3g; Sugar: 1g; Sodium: 86mg

Easy Baked Salmon

Servings: 4
Cooking Time: 16 Minutes
Ingredients:
- 4 salmon fillets
- 1 lemon zest
- 1 tsp sea salt
- 3 oz olive oil
- 1 garlic clove, minced
- 1 tsp fresh dill, chopped
- 1 tbsp fresh parsley, chopped
- 1/8 tsp white pepper

Directions:
1. Preheat the oven at 200°C.
2. Place all Ingredients: except salmon fillet in microwave safe bowl and microwave for 45 seconds.
3. Stir well until combine.
4. Place salmon fillets on parchment lined baking dish.
5. Spread evenly olive oil and herb mixture over each salmon fillet.
6. Place in preheated oven and bake for 15 minutes.
7. Serve and enjoy.

Nutrition:Per Servings: Calories: 40 Fat: 30.9 g, Carbohydrates: 0.5 g, Sugar: 0 g, Protein: 34.7 g, Cholesterol: 78 mg

Summer Breakfast Quinoa Bowls V

Servings: 2
Cooking Time: 30 Minutes
Ingredients:
- 1 sliced peach
- 1/3 c. Quinoa
- 1 c. Low fat milk
- ½ tsp. Vanilla extract
- 2 tsps. Natural stevia
- 12 raspberries
- 14 blueberries
- 2 tsps. Honey

Directions:
1. Add natural stevia, 2/3 cup milk and quinoa to a saucepan, and stir to combine.
2. Over medium high heat, bring to a boil then cover and reduce heat to a low simmer for a further minutes (you should be able to fluff quinoa with a fork).
3. Grease and preheat grill to medium. Grill peach slices for about a minute per side. Set aside.
4. Heat remaining milk in the microwave and set aside.
5. Split cooked quinoa evenly between 2 serving bowls and top evenly with remaining ingredients. Enjoy!

Nutrition: Calories: 180, Fat: 4g, Carbs: 3, Protein: 4.5g

Chocolate Overnight Oats

Servings: 2
Cooking Time: 5 Minutes

Ingredients:
- 1 tbsp unsweetened cocoa powder
- 1 cup rolled oats
- 1 cup unsweetened almond milk
- 1/4 tsp cinnamon
- 2/3 banana
- 2 tbsp walnuts, chopped

Directions:
1. Add banana in a medium bowl and mash using a fork.
2. Add cinnamon and cocoa powder and stir well.
3. Add almond milk and oats and stir to combine.
4. Cover and place in the refrigerator for overnight.
5. Stir oat mixture well. Top with walnuts and serve.

Nutrition:Per Servings: Calories 2 Fat 9.5 g Carbohydrates 40.2 g Sugar 5.4 g Protein 8.7 g Cholesterol 0 mg

Millet Congee

Servings: 4
Cooking Time: 60 Minutes
Ingredients:
- 1 cup millet
- 5 cups water
- 1 cup diced sweet potato
- 1 tsp. cinnamon
- 2 tbsps. stevia
- 1 diced apple
- ¼ cup honey

Directions:
1. In a deep pot, add stevia, sweet potato, cinnamon, water and millet, then stir to combine.
2. Bring to boil over high heat, then reduce to a simmer on low for an hour or until water is fully absorbed and millet is cooked.
3. Stir in remaining Ingredients: and serve.

Nutrition:Per Servings: Calories: 136, Fat: 1g, Carbs: 28.5g, Protein: 3.1g

Very Berry Muesli

Servings: 2
Cooking Time: 6 Hours
Ingredients:
- 1 c. Oats
- 1 c. Fruit flavored yogurt
- ½ c. Milk
- 1/8 tsp. Salt
- ½ c. Dried raisins
- ½ c. Chopped apple
- ½ c. Frozen blueberries
- ¼ c. Chopped walnuts

Directions:
1. Combine yogurt, salt and oats together in a medium bowl, mix well, then cover the mixture tightly.
2. Place in the refrigerator to cool for 6 hours.
3. Add raisins, and apples the gently fold.
4. Top with walnuts and serve. Enjoy!

Nutrition: Calories: 198, Carbs: 31.2g, Fat: 4.3g, Protein: 6g

Almond Oatmeal

Servings: 1
Cooking Time: 10 Minutes
Ingredients:
- 1/2 cup rolled oats
- 1 tbsp almond butter
- 1/2 cup unsweetened almond milk
- 1 tbsp cranberry sauce
- 1/4 tsp cinnamon
- 1/2 cup water

Directions:
1. Add oats, water, and almond milk in a small saucepan and cook over medium-high heat until thickened.
2. Remove from heat and add almond butter and cinnamon and stir well.
3. Top with cranberry sauce and serve.

Nutrition: Per Servings: Calories 278 Fat 13.g Carbohydrates 32.8 g Sugar 1.4 g Protein 9.3 g Cholesterol 0 mg

Hard-boiled Eggs And Avocado On Toast

Servings:4
Cooking Time: 10 Minutes
Ingredients:
- 4 eggs
- 4 slices sprouted whole-wheat bread, such as Angelic Bakehouse Sprouted Grain
- 1 medium avocado
- 1 teaspoon hot sauce
- Freshly ground black pepper
- Post-Op
- 1 toast

Directions:
1. Bring a large pot of water to a rapid boil over high heat.
2. Carefully add the eggs to the boiling water using a spoon, and set a timer for 10 minutes.

3. Immediately transfer the eggs from the boiling water to a strainer, and run cold water over the eggs to stop the cooking process.
4. Once the eggs are cool enough to handle, peel them and slice lengthwise into fourths.
5. Toast the bread.
6. While the bread toasts, mash the avocado with a fork in a small bowl and mix in the hot sauce.
7. Spread the avocado mash evenly across each toast. Top each toast slice with 4 egg slices and season with the black pepper.

Nutrition: Per Serving (1 toast): Calories: 191; Total fat: 10g; Protein: 10g; Carbs: 15g; Fiber: 5g; Sugar: 1g; Sodium: 214mg

Asparagus Omelet

Servings: 2
Cooking Time: 3 Minutes
Ingredients:
- 4 asparagus spears, peel lower half
- 4 tbsp parmesan cheese, grated
- 3 large eggs
- 2 tsp olive oil
- 1 garlic clove, minced
- Pepper
- Salt

Directions:
1. Heat olive oil in pan over medium heat.
2. Add asparagus and garlic in pan and sauté for 3 minutes.
3. Whisk together eggs, cheese, 1 tbsp water, pepper and salt.
4. Pour egg mixture over the asparagus and cook until desired doneness.
5. Serve and enjoy.

Nutrition: Per Servings: Calories: 159, Fat: 12.2 g, Carbohydrates: 3.0 g, Sugar: 1.5 g, Protein: 10.g, Cholesterol: 279 mg

Savory Parmesan Oatmeal

Servings: 1
Cooking Time: 35 Minutes
Ingredients:
- 1 - cup unsweetened almond milk
- 2/3 - cup rolled oats
- ½ - cup kale leaves, chopped
- ½ - cup broccoli florets, chopped
- Salt
- Pepper
- 1 - ounce parmesan, grated

Directions:
1. In a touch pot, warm temperature almond milk, 3 cup water, oats, kale, and broccoli. Season with salt and pepper.
2. Heat to the point of boiling, at that thing, decrease to stew and prepare dinner, blending at instances, till oats are whole, kale is withered, and broccoli is cooked although pretty company, 5 to 7minutes.
3. Top with parmesan.

Nutrition: Calories: 392;Carbs: g;Sugar: 3g;Protein: 21g

Perfect Granola

Servings: 10
Cooking Time: 40 Minutes
Ingredients:
- ¼ c. Canola oil
- 4 tbsps. Honey
- 1½ tsp. Vanilla
- 6 c. Old fashioned rolled oats
- 1 c. Almond
- ½ c. Shredded unsweetened coconut
- 2 c. Bran flakes
- ¾ c. Chopped walnuts
- 1 c. Raisins
- Cooking spray

Directions:
1. Prepare oven to preheat at 325 degrees f.
2. In a saucepan, cook oil and vanilla gently over low flame, occasionally stirring for roughly 5 mins.
3. Place all ingredients except raisins into a large bowl and combine.
4. Stir in honey and oil mixture slowly, ensuring all grains are properly coated.
5. Set a parchment paper on the baking tray or use cooking spray to grease lightly. Spread cereal evenly in the tray and bake for 2mins, occasionally stirring to keep mixture from burning, or until very lightly browned.
6. When ready, remove cereal and put aside to cool.
7. Add raisins and mix well.

Nutrition: Calories: 45 Fat: 21g, Carbs: 62g, Protein: 12.1g

High-protein Pancakes

Servings: 4
Cooking Time: 5 Minutes
Ingredients:
- 3 eggs
- 1 cup low-fat cottage cheese
- ⅓ cup whole-wheat pastry flour
- 1½ tablespoons coconut oil, melted
- Nonstick cooking spray
- Post-Op
- ½ pancake
- 1 to 2 pancakes

Directions:
1. In large bowl, lightly whisk the eggs.
2. Whisk in the cottage cheese, flour, and coconut oil just until combined.
3. Heat a large skillet or griddle over medium heat, and lightly coat with the cooking spray.
4. Using a measuring cup, pour ⅓ cup of batter into the skillet for each pancake. Cook for 2 to 3 minutes, or until bubbles appear across the surface of each pancake. Flip over the pancakes and cook for 1 to 2 minutes on the other side, or until golden brown.
5. Serve immediately.

Nutrition: Per Serving (1 pancake): Calories: 182; Total fat: 10g; Protein: 12g; Carbs: 10g; Fiber: 3g; Sugar: 1g; Sodium: mg

Smoothie Bowl With Greek Yogurt And Fresh Berries

Servings: 1
Cooking Time: 5 Minutes
Ingredients:
- ¾ cup unsweetened vanilla almond milk or low-fat milk
- ¼ cup low-fat plain Greek yogurt
- ⅓ cup (1 handful) fresh spinach
- ½ scoop (⅛ cup) plain or vanilla protein powder
- ¼ cup frozen mixed berries
- ¼ cup fresh raspberries
- ¼ cup fresh blueberries
- 1 tablespoon sliced, slivered almonds
- 1 teaspoon chia seeds
- Post-Op
- 1 bowl

Directions:
1. In a blender, combine the milk, yogurt, spinach, protein powder, and frozen berries. Blend on high speed for 3 to 4 minutes, until the powder is well dissolved and no longer visible.
2. Pour the smoothie into small bowl.
3. Decorate the smoothie with the fresh raspberries, blueberries, almonds, and chia seeds.
4. Serve with a spoon and enjoy!

Nutrition: Per Serving (1 bowl): Calories: 2; Total fat: 10 g; Protein: 20g; Carbs: 21g; Fiber: 8g; Sugar: 10g; Sodium: 262mg

Blackberry Almond Butter Sandwich

Servings: 1
Cooking Time: 0 Minutes
Ingredients:
- ¼ - cup blackberries
- 1 - teaspoon chia seeds
- 2 - slices 100-percent whole wheat bread, lightly toasted
- 2 - tablespoons natural almond butter

Directions:
1. In a bowl, pound blackberries softly with a fork. Mix in chia seeds.
2. Discretionary: cover and refrigerate blackberry-chia blend for as long as 4 days for a thick, jamlike consistency.
3. Collect sandwich with blackberry blend more than one cut of bread and almond margarine over another cut.

Nutrition: Calories: 5 Fat: 19g; Carbs: 52g ; Sugar 11g; Protein: 19g

Veggie Egg Scramble

Servings: 1
Cooking Time: 10 Minutes
Ingredients:
- 3 eggs, lightly beaten
- 1/4 cup bell peppers, chopped
- 4 mushrooms, chopped
- 1 tbsp olive oil
- 1/2 cup spinach, chopped
- Pepper
- Salt

Directions:
1. Heat 2 tablespoon of oil in a pan over medium heat.
2. Add vegetables and sauté for 5 minutes.
3. Heat remaining oil in another pan over medium heat.
4. Add eggs and stir until egg is scrambled and cooked, about 5 minutes. Season with pepper and salt.
5. Add sautéed vegetables in egg and stir well.
6. Serve and enjoy.

Nutrition: Per Servings: Calories 334 Fat 26 g Carbohydrates 6 g Sugar 3 g Protein 19 g Cholesterol 490 mg

Pumpkin Apple French Toast Bake

Servings: 3
Cooking Time: 40 Minutes
Ingredients:
- 6 - large eggs, ½ - cup canned pumpkin
- 2 - tablespoons almond butter
- 1 - tablespoon maple syrup
- 1 - teaspoon vanilla extract
- ½ - teaspoon cinnamon
- 4 - slices whole wheat bread, cut in 1-inch pieces
- 1 - medium apple, cored and very thinly sliced

Directions:
1. Warm broiler to 375°.
2. In a bowl, whisk eggs, pumpkin, almond margarine, maple syrup, vanilla, and cinnamon. Include bread and too until egg blend is ingested. Blend in apple.
3. Coat a little broiler-safe skillet (ideally cast iron) or 8-inch round cake container with cooking shower. Cautiously empty bread blend into skillet and press into an even layer.
4. Prepare until cooked through, puffed and marginally caramelized on top, 30 to 35 minutes. Cool somewhat before serving.
5. Cool remains totally before putting away in a water/air proof holder in the refrigerator.

Nutrition: Calories: 411; Carbs: 43g; Sugar: 1; Protein: 21g

Veggie Quiche Muffins

Servings: 12
Cooking Time: 50 Minutes
Ingredients:
- ¾ c. Shredded cheddar
- 1c. Green onion
- 1 c. Chopped broccoli
- 1 c. Diced tomatoes
- 2 c. Milk
- 4 eggs
- 1 c. Pancake mix
- 1 tsp. Oregano
- ½ tsp. Salt
- ½ tsp. Pepper

Directions:
1. Set oven to 375 degrees f, and lightly grease a cup muffin tin with oil.
2. Sprinkle tomatoes, broccoli, onions and cheddar into muffin cups.
3. Combine remaining ingredients in a medium bowl, whisk to combine then pour evenly on top of veggies.
4. Set to bake in preheated oven for about minutes or until golden brown.
5. Allow to cool slightly (about minutes) then serve. Enjoy!

Nutrition: Calories: 58.8, Fat: 3.2g, Carbs: 2.9g, Protein: 5.1g

Chocolate-peanut Butter French Toast

Servings: 1
Cooking Time: 0 Minutes
Ingredients:
- 1/3 - cup liquid egg whites
- 2 - teaspoons unsweetened cocoa powder
- ½ - teaspoon vanilla extract
- Salt
- 2 - slices whole-grain bread
- 1 - tablespoon peanut butter
- 2/3 - cup fresh raspberries

Directions:
1. In a shallow dish or bowl, whisk collectively egg whites, cocoa powder, vanilla, and a touch of salt. Absorb bread egg blend, each reduce in flip, until all the egg is ingested.
2. In a giant, nonstick skillet blanketed with cooking splash over medium warmth, consist of bread cuts and cook dinner till underside is dim brilliant darker, round 3minutes. Flip and cook until terrific darkish colored and marginally firm, round 3minutes greater.
3. Spread nutty unfold on French toast. Top with raspberries.

Nutrition: Calories 4; carbs 52g; protein 21g

Lunch and Dinner Recipes

Sheet Pan Zucchini Parmesan

Servings: 6
Cooking Time: 25 Minutes
Ingredients:
- 1 - cup panko
- 1/3 - cup freshly grated parmesan cheese
- Kosher salt and freshly ground black pepper, to taste
- 2 - zucchinis, thinly sliced to 1/4-inch thick rounds
- 1/3 - cup all-purpose flour
- 2 - large eggs, beaten
- ½ - cup marinara sauce
- ½ - cup mozzarella pearls, drained
- 2 - tablespoons chopped fresh parsley leaves

Directions:
1. Preheat broiler to 400 degrees f. Daintily oil a preparing sheet or coat with nonstick shower.
2. In an enormous bowl, consolidate panko and parmesan; season with salt and pepper, to taste. Put in a safe spot.
3. Working in clumps, dig zucchini adjusts in flour, dunk into eggs, at that point dig in panko blend, squeezing to cover.
4. Spot zucchini in a solitary layer onto the readied heating sheet. Spot into stove and heat until delicate and brilliant dark-colored, around 18 to 20 minutes.
5. Top with marinara and mozzarella.
6. At that point cook for 2 to 3minutes, or until the cheddar has dissolved.
7. Servings quickly, embellished with parsley, whenever wanted.
Nutrition: Calories: 217;carbs: 21g;fat: 12g;protein:

Grilled Fig And Peach Arugula Salad With Ricotta Salata And A Black Pepper Vinagretteprint

Servings:2
Cooking Time: 20 Minutes
Ingredients:
- Dressing:
- 3 - tablespoons good-quality olive oil
- 1 - teaspoon good balsamic vinegar
- ½ lemon from juice
- Salt
- 6 to 7 - turns freshly ground pepper
- Salad:
- 4 - figs, halved
- 1 - teaspoon dark brown sugar
- Salt
- Olive oil
- Few handfuls of arugulas, 2 ounces, cleaned and dried
- 1 - yellow peach, sliced
- 3 to 4 - pistachios, chopped
- 2 - slices prosciutto
- Ricotta salata

Directions:
1. In a little bowl, including the olive oil, balsamic vinegar, lemon juice, squeeze of salt and naturally ground pepper; blend until altogether joined. Do a trial and include more salt, in the event that you like. Put in a safe spot.
2. Sprinkle the figs with the dim dark colored sugar and a touch of salt. Warmth a barbecue or flame broil skillet. Whenever hot, brush with olive oil. Spot the figs on the hot flame broil, face down and cook for 1-minutes, until barbecue imprints show up. Expel and put in a safe spot.
3. To a huge blending bowl, include the arugula. Sprinkle the leaves with salt. Include half of the dressing and delicately prepare the serving of mixed greens. Move the lettuce to your serving plate. Add the peaches to the blending bowl and hurl with a touch of dressing. Move the peaches and figs to the serving plate, masterminding anyway you like. Top with a sprinkling of pistachios, a couple of torn bits of prosciutto and slight cuts of ricotta salata.
Nutrition: Calories: 3;carbs: 26g;fat: 24g;protein: 10g

Lean Spring Stew

Servings: 4
Cooking Time: 1 Hour 15 Minutes
Ingredients:
- 1 lb. diced fire roasted tomatoes
- 4 boneless, skinless chicken thighs
- 1 tbsp dried basil
- 8 oz chicken stock
- Salt & pepper to taste
- 4 oz tomato paste
- 3 chopped celery stalks
- 3 chopped carrots
- 2 chili peppers, finely chopped
- 2 tbsp olive oil
- 1 finely chopped onion
- 2 garlic cloves, crushed
- ½ container mushroomsSour cream

Directions:
1. Heat up the olive oil over medium-high temperature. Add the celery, onions and carrots and stir-fry for 5 to minutes.
2. Transfer to a deep pot and add tomato paste, basil, garlic, mushrooms and seasoning. Keep stirring the vegetables until they are completely covered by tomato sauce. At the same time, cut the chicken into small cubes to make it easier to eat.
3. Put the chicken in a deep pot, pour the chicken stock over it and throw in the tomatoes.
4. Stir the chicken in to ensure the ingredients and vegetables are properly mixed with it. Turn the heat to low and cook for about an hour. The vegetables and chicken should be cooked through before you turn the heat off. Top with sour cream and serve!

Nutrition:Per Serving: Net carbs 19 g;Fiber 3 g;Fats 11.9 g;Fatsr 3 g;Calories 277

Yummy Chicken Bites

Servings: 2
Cooking Time: 10 Minutes
Ingredients:
- 1 lb chicken breasts, skinless, boneless and cut into cubes
- 2 tbsp fresh lemon juice
- 1 tbsp fresh oregano, chopped
- 2 tbsp olive oil
- 1/8 tsp cayenne pepper
- Pepper
- Salt

Directions:
1. Place chicken in a bowl.
2. Add reaming ingredients over chicken and mix well.
3. Place chicken in the refrigerator for 1 hour.
4. Heat grill over medium heat.
5. Spray grill with cooking spray.
6. Thread marinated chicken onto skewers.
7. Arrange skewers on grill and grill until chicken is cooked.
8. Serve and enjoy.

Nutrition:Per Servings: Calories 560 Fat 31 g Carbohydrates 1.8 g Sugar 0.4 g Protein 66 g Cholesterol 200 mg

Shrimp Scampi

Servings: 4
Cooking Time: 10 Minutes

Ingredients:
- 1 lb. Shrimp
- 1/4 tsp red pepper flakes
- 1 tbsp fresh lemon juice
- 1/4 cup butter
- 1/2 cup chicken broth
- 2 garlic cloves, minced
- 1 shallot, sliced
- 3 tbsp olive oil
- 3 tbsp parsley, chopped
- Pepper
- Salt

Directions:
1. Heat oil in a pan over medium heat.
2. Add garlic and shallots and cook for 3 minutes.
3. Add broth, lemon juice, and butter and cook for 5 minutes.
4. Add red pepper flakes, parsley, pepper, and salt. Stir.
5. Add shrimp and cook for 3 minutes.
6. Serve and enjoy.

Nutrition: Calories 336;Fat 24 g;Carbohydrates 3 g;Sugar 0.2 g;Protein 26 g;Cholesterol 269 mg

Zucchini Frittata

Servings: 2
Cooking Time: 10 Minutes
Ingredients:
- 2 teaspoons butter (divided)
- 1 cup shredded zucchini
- Salt and freshly ground black pepper, to taste
- 4 eggs (lightly beaten)
- 2 tablespoons skim milk
- 1/4 teaspoon garlic salt
- 1/4 teaspoon onion powder
- 2 tablespoons shredded mild cheddar cheese

Directions:
1. In a medium nonstick skillet over medium heat, melt teaspoon butter and sauté zucchini until softened and lightly browned, 4 to 5 minutes, stirring frequently.
2. Drain zucchini if necessary and season to taste with salt and pepper. Beat eggs with milk, garlic salt, onion powder and zucchini until combined. Melt remaining 1 teaspoon butter in skillet, add egg mixture and cook until partially set. Lift edges of cooked egg with a spatula, let uncooked egg run underneath and continue until top of frittata is set, about 4 minutes.
3. Carefully flip frittata and let cook until lightly browned, to 4 minutes. Remove skillet from heat, sprinkle cheese over frittata and let stand until cheese is melted.
4. Cut frittata in half and serve immediately. Enjoy!

Nutrition:Per Serving: Calories: 20 Total Fat: 15g; Saturated Fat: 7g; Protein: 14g; Carbs: 4g; Fiber: 1g; Sugar: 3g

Salmon Patties

Servings: 3
Cooking Time: 10 Minutes
Ingredients:
- 14.5 oz can salmon
- 4 tbsp butter
- 1 avocado, diced
- 2 eggs, lightly beaten
- 1/2 cup almond flour
- 1/2 onion, minced
- Pepper
- Salt

Directions:
1. Add all ingredients except butter in a large mixing bowl and mix until well combined.
2. Make six patties from mixture. Set aside.
3. Melt butter in a pan over medium heat.
4. Place patties on pan and cook for 5 minutes on each side.
5. Serve and enjoy.

Nutrition: Calories 9;Fat 49 g;Carbohydrates 11 g;Sugar 2 g;Protein 36 g;Cholesterol 225 mg

Apple Cinnamon Oatmeal

Servings: 1
Cooking Time: 10 Minutes
Ingredients:
- 1/2 cup skim milk
- 1/3 cup water
- 1 apple (peeled, cored, diced)
- Dash of salt
- 1/2 cup old fashioned oats
- 1/4 teaspoon cinnamon
- 1/4 teaspoon vanilla

Directions:
1. Mix milk, water, apple and salt in a small saucepan and heat to a simmer, stirring occasionally (do not boil).
2. Add oats and cinnamon to saucepan and simmer, uncovered, for about 5 minutes, stirring occasionally.
3. Stir vanilla into oatmeal and serve immediately. Enjoy!

Nutrition:Per Serving: Calories: 18 Total Fat: 2g; Saturated Fat: 0g; Protein: 7g; Carbs: 36g; Fiber: 4g; Sugar: 19g

Stuff Cheese Pork Chops

Servings: 4
Cooking Time: 25 Minutes
Ingredients:
- 4 pork chops, boneless and thick cut
- 2 tbsp olives, chopped
- 2 tbsp sun-dried tomatoes, chopped
- ½ cup feta cheese, crumbled
- 2 garlic cloves, minced
- 2 tbsp fresh parsley, chopped

Directions:
1. Preheat the oven to 375 f.

2. In a bowl, mix together feta cheese, garlic, parsley, olives, and sun-dried tomatoes.
3. Stuff feta cheese mixture in the pork chops. Season with pepper and salt.
4. Bake for 35 minutes.
5. Serve and enjoy.

Nutrition: Calories 31Fat 25 g;Carbohydrates 2 g;Sugar 1 g;Protein 21 g;Cholesterol 75 mg

Italian Pork Chops

Servings: 4
Cooking Time: 30 Minutes
Ingredients:
- 4 pork loin chops, boneless
- 2 garlic cloves, minced
- 1 tsp Italian seasoning
- 1 tbsp fresh rosemary, chopped
- 1/4 tsp black pepper
- 1/2 tsp kosher salt

Directions:
1. Season pork chops with pepper and salt.
2. In a small bowl, mix together garlic, Italian seasoning, and rosemary.
3. Rub pork chops with garlic and rosemary mixture.
4. Place pork chops on a baking tray and roast in oven at 5 f for 10 minutes.
5. Turn temperature to 3 f and roast for 25 minutes more
6. Serve and enjoy.

Nutrition: Calories 261;Fat 19 g;Carbohydrates 2 g;Sugar 0 g;Protein 18 g;Cholesterol 68 mg;Fiber 0.4 g;Net carbs 1 g

Sunshine Wrap

Servings: 2
Cooking Time: 30 Minutes
Ingredients:
- 8 oz. Grilled chicken breast
- ½ c. Diced celery
- 2/3 c. Mandarin oranges
- ¼ c. Minced onion
- 2 tbsps. Mayonnaise
- 1 tsp. Soy sauce
- ¼ tsp. Garlic powder
- ¼ tsp. Black pepper
- 1 whole wheat tortilla
- 4 lettuce leaves

Directions:
1. Combine all ingredients, except tortilla and lettuce, in a large bowl and toss to evenly coat.
2. Lay tortillas on a flat surface and cut into quarters.
3. Top each quarter with a lettuce leaf and spoon chicken mixture into the middle of each.
4. Roll each tortilla into a cone and seal by slightly wetting the edge with water. Enjoy!

Nutrition: Calories: 280.8, Fat: 21.1g, Carbs: 3g, Protein: 19g

Taco Omelet

Servings: 1
Cooking Time: 10 Minutes
Ingredients:
- 2 eggs (lightly beaten)
- 2 tablespoons skim milk
- 1/4 teaspoon chili powder
- 1/4 teaspoon garlic powder
- 1/4 teaspoon onion powder
- Salt and freshly ground black pepper, to taste
- 1 teaspoon vegetable oil
- 1 tablespoon guacamole
- 1 tablespoon sour cream
- 1 tablespoon salsa
- 2 tablespoons shredded cojack cheese

Directions:
1. In a medium bowl, whisk eggs, milk, chili powder, garlic powder and onion powder and season to taste with salt and pepper.
2. Heat oil in a medium nonstick skillet over medium heat. Pour egg mixture into skillet and swirl to coat evenly. Cover skillet and let eggs cook until set on top, about 4 minutes.
3. With a large spatula, carefully flip omelet. Season omelet to taste with salt and pepper and let cook until lightly browned on the bottom, about minutes more.
4. Slide omelet onto a plate. Spread guacamole, sour cream and salsa all over one side of the omelet and sprinkle with cheese. Fold omelet in half over filling and serve immediately. Enjoy

Nutrition:Per Serving: Calories: 290; Total Fat: 22g; Saturated Fat: 10g; Protein: 17g; Carbs: 6g; Fiber: 1g; Sugar: 3g

Sheet Pan Spicy Tofu And Green Beans

Servings:4
Cooking Time: 30 Minutes
Ingredients:
- Spicy marinade:
- 1 - teaspoon minced garlic
- ¼ - cup sliced scallions
- 2 - teaspoons sesame seeds, plus more for garnish
- 3 - tablespoons soy sauce
- 1 - tablespoon sesame oil
- 1 - teaspoon red pepper flakes
- ½ - teaspoon maple syrup
- 2 - tablespoons of rice wine vinegar
- 16 - ounces firm tofu, drained and pressed
- 1 - pound green beans, trimmed
- 2 - teaspoons olive oil, for oiling the pan
- Salt/pepper

Directions:
1. Preheat the broiler to 400 degrees f.
2. Flush and channel your tofu, at that point press utilizing a tofu press or envelop by paper towels and spot overwhelming books or dish on top. Let channel for in any event 10 to 15 minutes, this will enable the marinade to be assimilated.
3. Whisk together the elements for the zesty sauce.

4. Cut the tofu into triangles and spot in a solitary layer on an oiled preparing sheet. Shower with the hot sauce at that point prepares for 12 minutes.
5. Flip tofu and sprinkle with more sauce. Add the green beans to the opposite side of the container in a solitary layer, as would be prudent. Shower with residual sauce and sprinkle with salt and pepper.
6. Return back to the stove and heat until tofu is caramelized and somewhat fresh, around 12-15 minutes.
7. Sprinkle with residual sesame seeds, whenever wanted, and serve.
Nutrition: Calories: 21carbs: 20g;fat: 11g;protein: 12g

Skillet Chicken Thighs With Potato, Apple, And Spinach

Servings:1
Cooking Time: 20 Minutes
Ingredients:
- 1 - small chicken thigh
- Salt
- Pepper
- 1 - teaspoon canola oil
- 1 - medium russet potato, cut into ½ inch cubes
- 1 - small fuji apple, cored and cut into 6 wedges
- 1 - teaspoon fresh sage, chopped
- 1 - cup packed baby spinach

Directions:
1. Warm broiler to 400°.
2. Season bird generously with salt and pepper.
3. In an extensive, broiler-secure skillet over medium warmth, warmness oil. Include bird, skin side down, and prepare dinner till pores and skin crisps marginally and a few fats are rendered round minutes. Include potato, apple, and sage. Toss to cowl and arrange potato and apple around the skillet, making sure hen is skin side down.
4. Move skillet to broiler and dish 15 minutes. Flip chicken, at that factor, broil 10 minutes extra, till potatoes and apples are delicate and chicken is cooked thru with no red within the middle.
5. Return skillet to stovetop over medium-low heat. Take off the chicken, consist of spinach and hurl with potatoes and apples to shrivel.
6. Top vegetable mixture with chook to serve.
Nutrition: Calories 514;fat 22g;carbs 59g;sugar 23g;protein 21g

Cherry Tomatoes Tilapia Salad

Servings: 3
Cooking Time: 25 Minutes
Ingredients:
- 1 c. Mixed greens
- 1 c. Cherry tomatoes
- ⅓ c. Diced red onion
- 1 medium avocado
- 3 tortilla crusted tilapia fillet

Directions:
1. Spray tilapia fillet with a little bit of cooking spray. Put fillets in air fryer basket. Cook for minutes at about 390° f.
2. Transfer the fillet to a bowl. Toss with tomatoes, greens and red onion. Add the lime dressing and mix again.
3. Serve and enjoy!
Nutrition: Calories: 271, fat: 8g, carbs: 10.1g, protein: 18.5g

Apple Cider Glazed Chicken Breast With Carrots

Servings: 2
Cooking Time: 6hrs 45 Minutes
Ingredients:
- 2 - boneless skin-on chicken breasts
- 2 - cups apple cider
- 4 - whole peppercorns
- 2 - small bunches of fresh sage
- ½ - teaspoon salt
- 2 - tablespoons olive oil
- Salt and pepper, to taste
- 4 - carrots, peeled and sliced
- 1 - tablespoon butter

Directions:
1. To start with, in all probability, your boneless skin-on chicken bosom still has the tenderloin connected. Expel (it's the additional piece that resembles a chicken strip). This helps the chicken cooks quicker. I solidify the tenderloins for soup or make chicken strips with them.
2. In an enormous dish or bowl, include the chicken, apple juice, peppercorns, sage (torn and hacked first), and ½ teaspoon of salt. Let marinate shrouded in the cooler for at least 4hrs.
3. Following 4hrs, expel the chicken and pat the chicken dry. Warm the oil in a huge skillet. At the point when the oil is hot, sprinkle the chicken with additional salt and pepper and spot its skin-side down in the container. Cook on both side until brilliant darker.
4. In the meantime, strip and bones the carrots. Spot them in a microwave-safe bowl, spread with saran wrap and microwave for 1 moment.
5. Take the flavors out from the apple juice, and after that pour it over the chicken once the two sides are brilliant dark colored. Change the warmth so the apple juice goes to a stew and cook until the chicken registers 16degrees f on a thermometer. Evacuate the chicken and put aside when done.
6. When the chicken is done, turn the warmth to high and lessen the apple juice to a thick coat. Include the carrots and saute for 3 to 4 minutes, until fresh delicate. Include the spread before

expelling them from the dish. Mix to cover the carrots in the coating and margarine. Utilize any additional coating from the dish to brush on the chicken and serve the chicken with the carrots.
Nutrition: Calories: 328;fat: 20g;carbs: 39g;sugar: 2;protein: 2g

Onion Paprika Pork Tenderloin

Servings: 6
Cooking Time: 30 Minutes
Ingredients:
- 2 lbs. Pork tenderloin
- For rub
- 1 1/2 tbsp smoked paprika
- 1 tbsp garlic powder
- 1 1/2 tbsp onion powder
- ½ tbsp salt

Directions:
1. Preheat the oven to 425 f.
2. In a small bowl, mix together all rub ingredients and rub over pork tenderloin.
3. Spray pan with cooking spray and heat over medium-high heat.
4. Sear pork on all sides until lightly golden brown.
5. Place pan into the oven and roast for about 230 minutes.
6. Sliced and serve.
Nutrition: Calories 225;Fat 5 g;Carbohydrates 2 g;Sugar 1 g;Protein 41 g;Cholesterol 45 mg

Rosemary Garlic Pork Chops

Servings: 4
Cooking Time: 35 Minutes
Ingredients:
- 4 pork chops, boneless
- ¼ tsp onion powder
- 2 garlic cloves, minced
- 1 tsp dried rosemary, crushed
- ¼ tsp pepper
- ¼ tsp sea salt

Directions:
1. Preheat the oven to 425 f.
2. Season pork chops with onion powder, pepper and salt.
3. Mix together rosemary and garlic and rub over pork chops.
4. Place pork chops on baking tray and roast for 10 minutes.
5. Set temperature 3 f and roast for 25 minutes more.
6. Serve and enjoy.
Nutrition: Calories 260;Fat 20 g;Carbohydrates 1 g;Sugar 0 g;Protein 19 g;Cholesterol mg

Skinny Chicken Pesto Bake

Servings: 4
Cooking Time: 35 Minutes
Ingredients:
- 160 oz. Skinless chicken
- 1 tsps. Basil
- 1 sliced tomato
- 6 tbsps. Shredded mozzarella cheese
- 2 tsps. Grated parmesan cheese

Directions:
1. Cut chicken into thin strips.
2. Set oven to 400 degrees f. Prepare a baking sheet by lining with parchment paper.
3. Lay chicken strips on prepared baking sheet. Top with pesto and brush evenly over chicken pieces.
4. Set to bake until chicken is fully cooked (about 15 minutes).
5. Garnish with parmesan cheese, mozzarella, and tomatoes.
6. Set to continue baking until cheese melts (about 5 minutes).

Nutrition: Calories: 205, fat: 8.5g, carbs: 2.5g, protein: 30g

Cold Tomato Couscous

Servings: 4
Cooking Time: 10 Minutes
Ingredients:
- 5 oz couscous
- 3 tbsp tomato sauce
- 3 tbsp lemon juice
- 1 small-sized onion, chopped
- 1 cup vegetable stock
- ½ small-sized cucumber, sliced
- ½ small-sized carrot, sliced
- ¼ tsp salt3 tbsp olive oil
- ½ cup fresh parsley, chopped

Directions:
1. First, pour the couscous into a large bowl. Boil the vegetable broth and slightly add in the couscous while stirring constantly. Leave it for about minutes until couscous absorbs the liquid. Cover with a lid and set aside. Stir from time to time to speed up the soaking process and break the lumps with a spoon.
2. Meanwhile, preheat the olive oil in a frying pan, and add the tomato sauce. Add chopped onion and stir until translucent. Set aside and let it cool for a few minutes.
3. Add the oily tomato sauce to the couscous and stir well. Now add lemon juice, chopped parsley, and salt to the mixture and give it a final stir.
4. Serve with sliced cucumber, carrot, and parsley.

Nutrition:Per Serving: Net carbs 32.8 g;Fiber 3.2 g;Fats 11 g;Fatsr 6 g;Calories 249

Cheesy Broccoli Soup

Servings: 4
Cooking Time: 20 Minutes
Ingredients:
- 2 teaspoons butter
- 1 tablespoon minced onion
- 1 garlic clove (minced)
- 3 cups chicken stock
- 4 cups broccoli florets
- Salt and freshly ground black pepper, to taste
- 2 cups skim milk
- 1/2 cup (about 2 ounces) shredded colby cheese

Directions:
1. In a large saucepan, melt butter and sauté onion until softened, about 5 minutes, stirring frequently. Add garlic and sauté about minute more, stirring constantly. Add chicken stock and broccoli to pan, season to taste with salt and pepper and heat to a boil. Cover pan, reduce heat and simmer until broccoli is softened, 10 to 15 minutes, stirring occasionally.
2. Add milk to soup and stir until heated through, 1 to minutes.
3. Remove pan from heat, add cheese and stir until cheese is melted. Serve soup immediately and enjoy!

Nutrition:Per Serving: Calories: 158; Total Fat: 7g; Saturated Fat: ; Protein: 11g; Carbs: 13g; Fiber: 2g; Sugar: 8g

Southwest Style Zucchini Rice Bowl

Servings: 2
Cooking Time: 12 Minutes
Ingredients:
- 1 tbsp. Vegetable oil
- 1 c. Chopped vegetables
- 1 c. Chopped chicken breast
- 1 c. Cooked zucchini rice
- 4 tbsps. Salsa
- 2 tbsps. Shredded cheddar cheese
- 2 tbsps. Sour cream

Directions:
1. Set a skillet with oil to heat up over medium heat.
2. Add chopped vegetables and allow to cook, stirring until vegetables become fork tender.
3. Add chicken and zucchini rice. Cook while stirring, until fully heated through.
4. Split between 2 serving bowls and garnish with remaining ingredients. Serve and enjoy!

Nutrition: Calories: 168, fat: 8.2g, carbs: 18g, protein: 5g

Creamy Salmon Salad

Servings: 2
Cooking Time: 5 Minutes
Ingredients:
- 6 oz can salmon, drained
- 1 celery stalk, sliced
- 1 avocado, chopped
- 1/2 bell pepper, chopped
- 2 tbsp low-fat yogurt
- 2 tbsp mustard
- 1/4 cup onion, minced

Directions:
1. In a mixing bowl, whisk together yogurt and mustard.
2. Add remaining ingredients and stir to combine.
3. Serve and enjoy.

Nutrition:Per Servings: Calories 5 Fat 27.8 g Carbohydrates 17.5 g Sugar 4.6 g Protein 24.3 g Cholesterol 34 mg

Dijon Chicken Thighs

Servings: 4
Cooking Time: 50 Minutes
Ingredients:
- 1 1/2 lbs chicken thighs, skinless and boneless
- 2 tbsp Dijon mustard
- 1/4 cup French mustard
- 2 tsp olive oil

Directions:
1. Preheat the oven to 375 F/ 0 C.
2. In a mixing bowl, mix together olive oil, Dijon mustard, and French mustard.
3. Add chicken to the bowl and mix until chicken is well coated.
4. Arrange chicken in a baking dish and bake for - 50 minutes.
5. Serve and enjoy.

Nutrition:Per Servings: Calories 348 Fat 15.2 g Carbohydrates 0.4 g Sugar 0.1 g Protein 49.g Cholesterol 151 mg

Buttery Shrimp

Servings: 4
Cooking Time: 15 Minutes
Ingredients:
- 1 1/2 lbs. Shrimp
- 1 tbsp Italian seasoning
- 1 lemon, sliced
- 1 stick butter, melted

Directions:
1. Add all ingredients into the large mixing bowl and toss well.
2. Transfer shrimp mixture on baking tray.
3. Bake at 0 f for 15 minutes.
4. Serve and enjoy.

Nutrition: Calories 41Fat 26 g;Carbohydrates 3 g;Sugar 0.3 g;Protein 39 g;Cholesterol 421 mg

Thyme Oregano Pork Roast

Servings: 6
Cooking Time: 1 Hour 40 Minutes
Ingredients:
- 3 lbs. Pork roast, boneless
- 1 cup chicken stock
- 1 onion, chopped
- 2 garlic cloves, chopped
- 1 rosemary sprig
- 3 fresh oregano sprigs
- 3 fresh thyme sprigs
- 1 tbsp pepper
- 1 tbsp olive oil
- 1 tbsp kosher salt

Directions:
1. Preheat the oven to 350 f.
2. Season meat with pepper and salt.
3. Heat olive oil in a stockpot and sear pork roast on each side, about 4 minutes on each side.
4. Add onion and garlic. Stir in the stock, oregano, and thyme and bring to boil for a minute.
5. Cover pot and roast in the preheated oven for 1 hour 30 minutes.
6. Serve and enjoy.

Nutrition:al value (per serving);Calories 501;Fat 24 g;Carbohydrates 3 g;Sugar 1 g;Protein 65 g;Cholesterol 194 mg

Honey & Soy Glazed Radishes

Servings: 2
Cooking Time: 15 Minutes
Ingredients:
- 1 - bunch of radishes, with greens
- 1 ½ - tablespoons olive oil
- ¼ - cup honey
- 2 - tablespoons soy sauce
- 1 - tablespoon unseasoned rice vinegar
- 1 - cup cooked white rice
- Fried eggs for serving

Directions:
1. Separate the greens from the radishes and generally slash them. Cut huge radishes into equal parts and keep littler radishes entirety.
2. Warm the oil in an enormous skillet over medium-high heat. Include the radishes and cook, blending frequently until daintily sautéed and fresh delicate, about 10 minutes. Include the nectar and lessen the warmth to medium. Cook, mixing regularly until the radishes are coated, around 3 to 5 minutes. Include the soy sauce and cook until syrupy, about 5 minutes longer. Blend in the rice vinegar and radish greens, increment the warmth to high and keep on cooking until the greens are shriveled and the vast majority of the fluid has vanished.
3. Present with cooked white rice and singed eggs.

Nutrition: Calories: 229;carbs: 2g;fat: 13g;protein: 2

Piña Colada Bark

Servings: 16
Cooking Time: 15 Minutes Plus 1 Hour
Refrigerating
Ingredients:
- 1/2 cup cocoa butter oil (melted)
- 1/2 cup coconut oil (melted)
- Powdered sweetener of choice equal to 2 tablespoons sugar
- 1 tablespoon pineapple extract
- 1 teaspoon coconut extract
- 1 teaspoon rum extract
- 1/2 cup unsweetened shredded coconut (toasted)

Directions:
1. Line an 8" x 8" baking pan with aluminum foil and set aside.
2. In a medium bowl, mix cocoa butter, coconut oil, sweetener and extracts until thoroughly combined.
3. Pour mixture into prepared pan, spread evenly and sprinkle with coconut. Cover pan with plastic wrap and refrigerate until bark is chilled through and firm, about 1 hour.
4. Use foil to lift bark from pan. Cut bark into 16 squares and serve immediately. Enjoy!

Nutrition:Per Serving: Calories: 137; Total Fat: 1; Saturated Fat: 10g; Protein: 0g; Carbs: 2g; Fiber: 0g; Sugar: 0g

Rosemary Garlic Pork Roast

Servings: 6
Cooking Time: 1 Hour 10 Minutes
Ingredients:
- 4 lbs. Pork loin roast, boneless
- 4 garlic cloves, peeled
- 2 lemon juice
- 1/4 cup fresh sage leaves
- 1/3 cup fresh rosemary leaves
- 1 tbsp salt

Directions:
1. Add sage, rosemary, garlic, lemon juice, and salt into the blender and blend until smooth.
2. Rub herb paste all over roast and place on hot grill.
3. Grill for 1 hour.
4. Sliced and serve.

Nutrition: Calories 6;Fat 30 g;Carbohydrates 5 g;Sugar 1 g;Protein 88 g;Cholesterol 246 mg

Cottage Cheese Pancakes

Servings: 4
Cooking Time: 10 Minutes
Ingredients:
- 1 cup low-fat cottage cheese
- 3 eggs (lightly beaten)
- 1 1/2 teaspoons vegetable oil
- 1/2 cup flour
- 1/2 teaspoon baking powder

Directions:
1. For the batter, whisk cottage cheese, eggs and oil until thoroughly combined. Toss flour and baking powder and stir into cottage cheese mixture just until combined.
2. Spray a large nonstick skillet with cooking spray and heat over medium heat. Pour batter in 1/cup portions into skillet and fry until bubbly on top, 3 to 4 minutes. Flip pancakes and cook until browned and cooked through, 2 to 3 minutes more.
3. Serve pancakes as desired and enjoy!

Nutrition:Per Serving: Calories: 171; Total Fat: 6g; Saturated Fat: 2g; Protein: 1; Carbs: 14g; Fiber: 0g; Sugar: 1g

Herb Pork Chops

Servings: 4
Cooking Time: 30 Minutes
Ingredients:
- 4 pork chops, boneless
- 1 tbsp olive oil
- 2 garlic cloves, minced
- 1 tsp dried rosemary, crushed
- 1 tsp oregano
- ½ tsp thyme
- 1 tbsp fresh rosemary, chopped
- ¼ tsp pepper
- ¼ tsp salt

Directions:
1. Preheat the oven 425 f.
2. Season pork chops with pepper and salt and set aside.
3. In a small bowl, mix together garlic, oil, rosemary, oregano, thyme, and fresh rosemary and rub over pork chops.
4. Place pork chops on baking tray and roast for 10 minutes.
5. Turn heat to 3 f and roast for 25 minutes more.
6. Serve and enjoy.

Nutrition: Calories 260;Fat 22 g;Carbohydrates 2.5 g;Sugar 0 g;Protein 19 g;Cholesterol 65 mg

Mayo-less Tuna Salad

Servings: 2
Cooking Time: 5 Minutes
Ingredients:
- 5 oz. Tuna
- 1 tbsp. Olive oil
- 1 tbsp. Red wine vinegar
- ¼ c. Chopped green onion
- 2 c. Arugula
- 1 c. Cooked pasta
- 1 tbsp. Parmesan cheese
- Black pepper

Directions:
1. Combine all ingredients into a medium bowl. Split mixture between two plates. Serve, and enjoy.

Nutrition: Calories: 3.2, Fat: 6.2g, Carbs: 20.3g, Protein: 22.7g

Stuffed Omelet With Almonds

Servings: 2
Cooking Time: 15 Minutes
Ingredients:
- 2 tablespoons sliced almonds
- 4 eggs (lightly beaten)
- 2 tablespoons skim milk
- 1 teaspoon butter
- 1/2 cup low-fat cottage cheese
- Salt and freshly ground black pepper, to taste

Directions:
1. In a medium dry nonstick skillet over medium heat, toast almonds until lightly browned, stirring occasionally, 4 to 5 minutes. Remove almonds from skillet and set aside.
2. Whisk eggs and milk until thoroughly combined and season to taste with salt and pepper. Melt butter in the same skillet and pour in eggs. When eggs begin to cook, gently lift the cooked edges and tilt skillet to allow uncooked eggs to flow underneath. Continue lifting and tilting all around until no uncooked eggs remain on top of the cooked portion.
3. Cover skillet and let cook until omelet is lightly browned on the bottom, 2 to minutes. Carefully flip omelet and cook until lightly browned, 3 to 4 minutes.
4. Slide omelet out of pan onto a serving plate and season to taste with salt and pepper. Spread cottage cheese over half of the omelet and sprinkle with toasted almonds. Fold omelet over filling , cut in half and serve immediately. Enjoy!
Nutrition:Per Serving: Calories: 234; Total Fat: 1; Saturated Fat: 5g; Protein: 21g; Carbs: 5g; Fiber: 1g; Sugar: 2g

Savory Stuffed Crepes

Servings: 4
Cooking Time: 15 Minutes
Ingredients:
- 2 tablespoons butter (divided)
- 2 scallions (sliced)
- 1 garlic clove (minced)
- 1 package (3 ounces) cream cheese (softened)
- 1 tablespoon sour cream
- 4 eggs
- 1/2 cup skim milk
- 1/4 cup flour
- Salt and freshly ground black pepper, to taste

Directions:
1. For the filling, heat tablespoon butter in a small nonstick skillet and sauté scallions until softened, about 2 minutes, stirring occasionally. Add garlic and sauté about 1 minute more, stirring constantly. Mix cream cheese and sour cream until smooth, add scallion mixture and stir until combined. Set filling aside.
2. For the crepes, whisk eggs, milk and flour in a medium bowl and season to taste with salt and pepper. Melt remaining 1 tablespoon butter in a medium nonstick skillet over medium heat and fry portions of egg mixture into 4 crepes.
3. Spread about 1/4 of the filling up the center of each crepe and roll up crepes to cover filling. Serve immediately and enjoy!
Nutrition:Per Serving: Calories: 238; Total Fat: 18G; Saturated Fat: 10g; Protein: 9g; Carbs: 9g; Fiber: 0g; Sugar: 2g

Crab Cakes

Servings: 4
Cooking Time: 15 Minutes
Ingredients:
- 1 egg
- 2 tbsp butter
- 1 tbsp cilantro, chopped
- 1/2 cup almond flour
- 4 tbsp pork rinds
- 1 lb. Crab meat
- 3 tsp ginger garlic paste
- 2 tsp sriracha
- 2 tsp lemon juice
- 1 tsp Dijon mustard
- 1/4 cup mayonnaise

Directions:
1. Add all ingredients except butter in a large bowl and mix until well combined.
2. Preheat the oven to 350 f.
3. Heat butter in a pan over medium-high heat.
4. Make crab cake from mixture and place in the pan and cook for 5 minutes.
5. Transfer pan in preheated oven and bake for 10 minutes.
6. Serve and enjoy.
Nutrition: Calories 251;Fat 16 g;Carbohydrates 4 g;Sugar 0.9 g;Protein 15 g;Cholesterol 97 mg

Sheet Pan Garlic Tofu & Brussels Sprout Dinner

Servings: 4
Cooking Time: 30 Minutes
Ingredients:
- 14 - ounce package of extra firm organic tofu, pressed
- 1 - pound brussels sprouts, cleaned and diced, approximately 2 cups prepared 1 - tablespoon olive oil
- 2 - tablespoon balsamic vinegar
- 1 - tablespoon minced garlic
- ¼ - teaspoon sea salt
- ¼ - teaspoon black pepper
- ½ - cup dried cranberries
- ¼ - cup pumpkin seeds
- 1 - tablespoon balsamic glaze

Directions:
1. Preheat the broiler to 400 degrees f
2. Channel the overabundance water from the holder of tofu.
3. Shakers the tofu into 1-inch reduced down pieces and press between two clean towels for 15 minutes to wick away extra dampness.
4. Reap, clean and bones your brussels grows.
5. In a big bowl, combine the brussels grows, oil, vinegar, and garlic. Include the salt, pepper, and tofu and big tenderly until the tofu is all around covered.
6. Splash a foil-fixed heating sheet with cooking shower.
7. Put into the stove and heat for 20 minutes.
8. After 20 minutes, expel from the stove and blend.
9. Equally spread the pumpkin seeds and cranberries and come back to the broiler for an extra 10 minutes.
10. Take out from the stove and sprinkle with balsamic coating.
Nutrition: Calories: 250; fat: 2g; carbs: 18g; sugar: 13g; protein: 13g

Huevos Rancheros

Servings: 2
Cooking Time: 15 To 20 Minutes
Ingredients:
- 1 can (14 ounces) diced tomatoes with green chilies
- 1 teaspoon chili powder, plus more if desired
- 1/2 teaspoon onion powder
- 1/2 teaspoon garlic powder
- 4 eggs
- Salt and freshly ground black pepper, to taste

Directions:
1. For the sauce, mix undrained tomatoes, chili powder, onion powder and garlic powder in a medium nonstick skillet over medium heat and season to taste with salt and pepper. Heat tomato mixture to a boil, reduce heat, cover and simmer for about 5 minutes.
2. Make 4 wells in the tomato mixture. Crack an egg into a small bowl and pour into one of the wells. Repeat with remaining eggs. Sprinkle more chili powder over eggs if desired.
3. Cover skillet and simmer until eggs are cooked to desired consistency; about 5 minutes for soft and runny yolks, up to 10 minutes for firm and hard yolks.
4. Scoop eggs onto plates and top with the sauce to serve. Enjoy!
Nutrition:Per Serving: Calories: 166; Total Fat: 9g; Saturated Fat: 3g; Protein: 13g; Carbs: 10g; Fiber: 1g; Sugar: 1g

Nutty Chocolate Bites

Servings: 12
Cooking Time: 15 Minutes Plus 30 Minutes Freezing
Ingredients:
- 1/2 cup coconut oil (melted)
- 1/4 cup smooth natural peanut butter (melted)
- 1 tablespoon butter (melted)
- 2 tablespoons unsweetened cocoa powder (sifted)
- 1/4 cup chopped roasted peanuts

Directions:
1. Line wells of a mini muffin pan with paper liners and set aside.
2. In a small bowl, beat coconut oil, peanut butter and butter with an electric hand mixer until smooth and thoroughly combined.
3. Sprinkle cocoa powder over coconut oil mixture and continue beating until smooth and thoroughly combined.
4. Pour mixture into prepared pan and sprinkle with chopped peanuts. Place muffin pan in the freezer until cups are firm and chilled through, about 30 minutes. Serve and enjoy!
Nutrition:Per Serving: Calories: 136; Total Fat: 14g; Saturated Fat: 9g; Protein: 2g; Carbs: 2g; Fiber: 1g; Sugar: 1g

Pesto & Mozzarella Stuffed Portobello Mushroom Caps

Servings: 2
Cooking Time: 30 Minutes
Ingredients:
- 2 portobello mushrooms
- 1 diced roma tomato
- 2 tbsps. Pesto
- ¼ c. Shredded mozzarella cheese

Directions:
1. Spoon pesto evenly into mushroom caps, then top with remaining ingredients. Bake at 400 degrees f for about minutes. Enjoy!
Nutrition: Calories: 11 fat: 5.4g, carbs: 7.5g, protein: 10.5g

Vegetables In Wok

Servings: 4
Cooking Time: 20 Minutes
Ingredients:
- 1 lb. chicken breast, boneless and skinless
- 1 medium red pepper, cut into strips
- 1 medium green pepper, cut into strips
- 7-8 pieces baby corn
- ½ cup canned button mushroom
- s1 cup cauliflower
- 1 medium carrot, peeled and cut into strips
- 1 tsp tomato sauce, sugar-free
- Salt to taste
- 1 tbsp olive oil

Directions:
1. Cut the meat into bite size pieces.
2. In a large wok, heat up the olive oil over a high temperature. Add the chicken meat and cook for about 10 minutes, stirring constantly.
3. Remove from the wok. Now cook the vegetables by first adding carrot strips and cauliflower. They take the most time to soften. Then add red and green pepper strips, baby corn, button mushrooms, and tomato sauce.
4. Cook for another 5-7 minutes. You don't want to overcook the vegetables. They have to stay crispy.
5. Add the meat, mix well and serve with rice.

Nutrition:Per Serving: Net carbs 57.g;Fiber 9.4 g;Fats 9.7 g;Fatsr 2 g;Calories 420

Beef Roast With Winter Vegetables

Servings: 6
Cooking Time: 3 Hours
Ingredients:
- 2 - lb. Chuck or round roast
- 2 - cups baby carrots or carrot sticks
- 2 - large parsnips, peeled and cut into chunks
- 4 - medium sweet potatoes
- 1 - acorn squash, peeled, seeded and cubed
- 1 - teaspoon Italian seasoning
- Drizzles of olive oil and balsamic vinegar
- Salt and pepper, to taste

Directions:
1. Preheat the broiler to 400 f.
2. Spot the hamburger cook in the focal point of a medium-sized broiling container. Toss the carrots, parsnips, sweet potatoes, and squash around the hamburger cook. Season with Italian flavoring at that point showers olive oil and balsamic vinegar over the top.
3. Spread the cooking container and spot in the preheated broiler. Cook for around two hours, contingent upon the size of the meal.
4. Addition a meat thermometer and cook until 1 f for medium to 165 f for all-around done.
5. In the event that you favor a juicier, however, less crusted dish, cook it at 32f for around three hours, or until the meat thermometer peruses 145 f, for medium-well.
6. Servings hamburger cook with winter vegetables as may be, or with a straightforward side plate of mixed greens.

Nutrition: Calories: 295;carbs: 28g;fat: 1;protein: 3g

Carrot Sweet Potato Soup

Servings: 4

Cooking Time: 8 Minutes
Ingredients:
- 1 lb. sweet potato, peeled and cut into chunks
- 1/2 lb. carrots, chopped
- 1 tbsp olive oil
- 1 tbsp ginger, grated
- 6 cups vegetable broth
- Pepper
- Salt

Directions:
1. Heat oil in a saucepan over medium heat.
2. Add carrots and sweet potato and sauté for 10 minutes.
3. Add ginger and cook for 2 minutes.
4. Add broth and stir well. Bring to boil.
5. Turn heat to low and simmer for 20 minutes.
6. Remove pan from heat. Puree the soup using an immersion blender until smooth.
7. Season with pepper and salt.
8. Serve and enjoy.

Nutrition: Calories 218;Fat 5.8 g;Carbohydrates 31.4 g;Sugar 11.2 g;Protein 10.g;Cholesterol 0 mg

Lemon Pepper Pork Tenderloin

Servings: 4
Cooking Time: 25 Minutes
Ingredients:
- 1 lb. Pork tenderloin
- 3/4 tsp lemon pepper
- 1 1/2 tsp dried oregano
- 1 tbsp olive oil
- 4 tbsp feta cheese, crumbled
- 2 1/2 tbsp olive tapenade

Directions:
1. Add pork, oil, lemon pepper, and oregano in a zip-lock bag. Seal bag and rub well and place in a refrigerator for 2 hours.
2. Remove pork from zip-lock bag.
3. Using a sharp knife make lengthwise cut through the center of the tenderloin.
4. Spread olive tapenade on half tenderloin and sprinkle with crumbled cheese.
5. Fold another half of meat over to the original shape of tenderloin.
6. Close pork tenderloin with twine at 2-inch intervals.
7. Grill for 20 minutes. Turn tenderloin during grilling.
8. Sliced and serve.

Nutrition: Calories 215;Fat 10 g;Carbohydrates 1 g;Sugar 1 g;Protein 31 g;Cholesterol mg

Roasted Parmesan Cauliflower

Servings: 4
Cooking Time: 30 Minutes
Ingredients:
- 8 cups cauliflower florets
- 1 tsp Italian seasoning, crushed
- 2 tbsp olive oil
- 1/2 cup parmesan cheese, shredded
- 2 tbsp balsamic vinegar
- 1/4 tsp pepper
- 1/4 tsp salt

Directions:
1. Preheat the oven to 450 F/ 232 C.
2. Toss cauliflower, Italian seasoning, oil, pepper, and salt in a bowl.
3. Spread cauliflower on a baking tray and roast for 15-20 minutes.
4. Toss cauliflower with cheese and vinegar.
5. Return to the oven and roast for 10 minutes more.
6. Serve and enjoy.

Nutrition: Calories 196;Fat 13 g;Carbohydrates 12 g;Sugar 4 g;Protein 11 g;Cholesterol 14 mg

Delicious Chicken Salad

Servings: 4
Cooking Time: 5 Minutes
Ingredients:
- 1 lb. cooked chicken breasts, diced
- 1/2 cup olives, sliced
- 1 tbsp capers
- 2 tbsp olive oil
- 2 tbsp vinegar
- 1/2 cup onion, minced
- 2 tbsp fresh parsley, chopped
- 1 tbsp fresh basil, chopped
- 1/4 tsp chili flakes
- Salt

Directions:
1. Add all ingredients into the mixing bowl and toss well.
2. Serve and enjoy.

Nutrition: Calories 5;Fat 18 g;Carbohydrates 3.2 g;Sugar 1 g;Protein 33 g;Cholesterol 100 mg

Baked Salmon

Servings: 4
Cooking Time: 35 Minutes
Ingredients:
- 1 lb. Salmon fillet
- 4 tbsp parsley, chopped
- 1/4 cup mayonnaise
- 1/4 cup parmesan cheese, grated
- 2 garlic cloves, minced
- 2 tbsp butter

Directions:
1. Preheat the oven to 350 f.
2. Place salmon on greased baking tray.
3. Melt butter in a pan over medium heat.

4. Add garlic and sauté for minute.
5. Add remaining ingredient and stir to combined.
6. Spread pan mixture over salmon fillet.
7. Bake for 20-25 minutes.
8. Serve and enjoy.

Nutrition: Calories 412;Fat 26 g;Carbohydrates 4.3 g;Sugar 1 g;Protein 34 g;Cholesterol mg

Nutty Crunch Porridge

Servings: 1
Cooking Time: 10 Minutes
Ingredients:
- 1 cup almond milk
- 3 tablespoons farina breakfast porridge mix (such as Cream of Wheat or Malt-O-Meal)
- Dash of salt
- 1 tablespoons sliced almonds (toasted)

Directions:
1. In a small saucepan, heat almond milk to a simmer (do not boil).
2. Whisk farina into milk until smooth.
3. Reduce heat and simmer, uncovered, until porridge is thickened, about 2 minutes, stirring occasionally.
4. Stir salt into porridge. Pour porridge into a bowl and sprinkle with almonds to serve. Enjoy!

Nutrition:Per Serving: Calories: 1; Total Fat: 11g; Saturated Fat: 1g; Protein: 5g; Carbs: 10g; Fiber: 3g; Sugar: 1g

Creamy Cauliflower Soup

Servings: 4
Cooking Time: 20 Minutes
Ingredients:
- 1/2 head cauliflower, diced
- 1 small onion, diced
- 1 tbsp olive oil
- 1 garlic clove, minced
- 15 oz vegetable broth
- 1/2 tsp salt

Directions:
1. Heat olive oil in a saucepan over medium heat.
2. Add onion and garlic and sauté for 5 minutes.
3. Add cauliflower and broth. Stir well and bring to boil.
4. Cover and simmer for 15 minutes. Season with salt.
5. Puree the soup using an immersion blender until smooth.
6. Serve and enjoy.

Nutrition: Calories 41;Fat 1.5 g;Carbohydrates 4.1 g;Sugar 2 g;Protein 3.2 g;Cholesterol 0 mg

Chili Garlic Salmon

Servings: 3
Cooking Time: 2 Minutes
Ingredients:
- 1 lb salmon fillet, cut into three pieces
- 1 tsp red chili powder
- 1 garlic clove, minced
- 1 tsp ground cumin
- Pepper
- Salt

Directions:
1. Pour 1/2 cups water into the instant pot and place trivet into the pot.
2. In a small bowl, mix together chili powder, garlic, cumin, pepper, and salt.
3. Rub salmon pieces with spice mixture and place on top of the trivet.
4. Seal the instant pot with a lid and cook on steam mode for 2 minutes.
5. Once done, release pressure using the quick-release method than open the lid.
6. Serve and enjoy.

Nutrition:Per Servings: Calories 205 Fat 9 g Carbohydrates 1.1 g Sugar 0.1 g Protein 30 g Cholesterol 65 mg

Chicken Chili Recipe For One

Servings: 1
Cooking Time: 35 Minutes
Ingredients:
- 1 - tablespoon olive oil
- 1 - cup chopped onion (1/2 small onion)
- 1 - garlic clove, minced
- 1 - small red pepper, cored, seeded, and large diced
- ¼ - teaspoon chili powder
- ¼ - teaspoon ground cumin
- ½ - teaspoon kosher salt
- 1 15 - ounce can of diced tomatoes
- ½ - teaspoon dried basil
- 1 - chicken breast, cooked and chopped
- Shredded cheddar cheese, optional for topping
- Sour cream, optional for topping

Directions:
1. Cook the onions inside the olive oil over medium-low warmness for 8 to minutes, till the onions are translucent.
2. Add the garlic and cook for 1 minute more.
3. Add the pink peppers, chili powder, cumin, and salt. Cook for 1mint
4. Pour the canned diced tomatoes and dried basil into the pan. Bring to a boil, and then lessen warmth to low and simmer, exposed for 15 minutes.
5. Add the cooked, chopped hen to the pan and simmer, exposed another minutes.
6. Transfer chicken chili to a bowl and top with shredded cheddar cheese and sour cream.

Nutrition: Calories: 4kcal;carbs: 21g;protein: 50g;fat: 20g;sugar: 9g.

Spaghetti Squash Lasagna

Servings: 6
Cooking Time: 30 Minutes
Ingredients:
- 2 cup marinara sauce
- 3 cup roasted spaghetti squash
- 1 cup ricotta
- 8 tsps. grated parmesan cheese
- 6 oz. shredded mozzarella cheese
- ¼ tsp. red pepper flakes

Directions:
1. Set oven to preheat oven to 375 degrees F and spoon half of marinara sauce into baking dish.
2. Top with squash, then layer remaining Ingredients:.
3. Cover and set to bake until cheese is melted and edges brown (about 20 minutes).
4. Remove cover and return to bake for another 5 minutes. Enjoy!

Nutrition:Per Servings: Calories: 2, Fat: 15.9g , Carbs: 5.5g, Protein: 21.4g

Crab Mushrooms

Servings: 5
Cooking Time: 20 Minutes
Ingredients:
- 5 oz. Crab meat
- 5 oz. White mushrooms
- ½ tsp. Salt
- ¼ c. Fish stock
- 1 tsp. Butter
- ¼ tsp. Ground coriander
- 1 tsp. Dried cilantro
- 1 tsp. Butter

Directions:
1. Chop the crab meat and sprinkle with salt and dried cilantro.
2. Mix the crab meat carefully. Preheat the air fryer to 400 f.
3. Chop the white mushrooms and combine with crab meat.
4. Add fish stock, ground coriander and butter.
5. Transfer the side dish mixture into the air fryer basket tray.
6. Stir gently with the help of a plastic spatula.
7. Cook the side dish for 5 minutes.
8. Rest for 5 minutes. Serve and enjoy!

Nutrition: Calories: 56, fat: 1.7g, carbs: 2.6g, protein: 7g

Cauliflower Mushroom Soup

Servings: 4
Cooking Time: 26 Minutes
Ingredients:
- 1 1/2 cup mushrooms, diced
- 2 cups cauliflower florets
- 1/2 onion, diced
- 1 tsp onion powder
- 1 2/3 cup coconut milk
- 1/2 tbsp olive oil
- 1/4 tsp pepper
- 1/4 tsp salt

Directions:
1. Add cauliflower, coconut milk, onion powder, pepper, and salt in a saucepan. Bring to boil over medium heat.
2. Turn heat to low and simmer for 8 minutes.
3. Puree the soup using an immersion blender until smooth.
4. Heat oil in another saucepan over high heat.
5. Add onion and mushrooms and sauté for 8 minutes.
6. Add cauliflower mixture to sautéed mushrooms. Stir well and bring to boil.
7. Cover and simmer for 10 minutes.
8. Serve and enjoy.

Nutrition: Calories 260;Fat 24 g;Carbohydrates 11 g;Sugar 5 g;Protein 4 g;Cholesterol 0 mg

One Pan Parmesan-crusted Chicken With Broccoli

Servings: 6
Cooking Time: 30 Minutes
Ingredients:
- 2 - tablespoons olive oil
- ½ - cup freshly grated parmesan cheese
- 6 to 7- ounce boneless, skinless chicken breasts
- 1 - teaspoon kosher salt
- 12 - ounces fresh or frozen broccoli florets
- 2 - garlic cloves, minced
- ¼ - tsp garlic powder
- ¼ - cup chopped fresh parsley

Directions:
1. Preheat the broiler to 425°f. Oil a rimmed preparing sheet with tablespoon of the olive oil.
2. Organize the chicken bosoms in the focal point of the readied preparing sheet. Orchestrate the broccoli around the chicken.
3. Shower the broccoli with the staying 1 tablespoon olive oil and sprinkle everything with salt and garlic powder.
4. Prepare until the chicken bosoms are cooked through and a thermometer embedded in the thickest part enlists 160°f, 25 to 30 minutes.
5. In a little bowl, consolidate the garlic, parmesan, and parsley.
6. Top every chicken bosom with a portion of the blends. Sear until the cheddar is softened and the broccoli is profoundly cooked 3minutes.
7. Take the container out from the broiler, tent with foil, and let rest for 5 minutes. Servings warm.

Nutrition: Calories: 334;carbs: 4g;fat: 13g;protein: 51g

Baked Lemon Tilapia

Servings: 4

Cooking Time: 12 Minutes
Ingredients:
- 4 tilapia fillets
- 2 tbsp fresh lemon juice
- 1 tsp garlic, minced
- 1/4 cup olive oil
- 2 tbsp fresh parsley, chopped
- 1 lemon zest
- Pepper
- Salt

Directions:
1. Preheat the oven to 425 F/ 220 C.
2. Spray a baking dish with cooking spray and set aside.
3. In a small bowl, whisk together olive oil, lemon zest, lemon juice, and garlic.
4. Season fish fillets with pepper and salt and place in the baking dish.
5. Pour olive oil mixture over fish fillets.
6. Bake fish fillets in the oven for 10-12 minutes.
7. Garnish with parsley and serve.

Nutrition:Per Servings: Calories 252 Fat 14.7 g Carbohydrates 0.5 g Sugar 0.2 g Protein 32.2 g Cholesterol mg

Delicious Seafood Dip

Servings: 16
Cooking Time: 30 Minutes
Ingredients:
- 1/2 lb. Shrimp, cooked
- 4 oz can green chilies
- 2 cups pepper jack cheese
- 4 oz cream cheese
- 1/2 tsp old bay seasoning
- 2 garlic cloves, minced
- 1/2 cup spinach, minced
- 1/2 cup onion, minced
- 2 tbsp butter
- 4 oz crab meat

Directions:
1. Preheat the oven to 425 f.
2. Melt butter in a pan over medium heat.
3. Add garlic, old bay seasoning, spinach, crab meat, chilies, and shrimp and cook for 4-5 minutes.
4. Add 1 cup pepper jack cheese and cream cheese.
5. Top with remaining cheese and bake for 20 minutes.
6. Serve and enjoy.

Nutrition: Calories 63;Fat 4 g;Carbohydrates 1 g;Sugar 0.2 g;Protein 5 g;Cholesterol 45 mg

Shrimp & Broccoli

Servings: 2
Cooking Time: 7 Minutes
Ingredients:
- 1/2 lb. Shrimp
- 1 tsp fresh lemon juice
- 2 tbsp butter
- 2 garlic cloves, minced
- 1 cup broccoli florets
- Salt

Directions:
1. Melt butter in a pan over medium heat.
2. Add garlic and broccoli to pan and cook for 3-4 minutes.
3. Add shrimp and cook for 4 minutes.
4. Add lemon juice and salt and stir well.
5. Serve and enjoy.

Nutrition: Calories 257;Fat 13 g;Carbohydrates g;Sugar 0.9 g;Protein 27 g;Cholesterol 269 mg

Spicy Tofu Quinoa Bowls

Servings: 4
Cooking Time: 45 Minutes
Ingredients:
- 1 package (15 ounces) extra-firm tofu
- 2 tablespoons soy sauce
- 1 teaspoon sesame oil
- Salt and freshly ground black pepper, to taste
- 1 cup uncooked quinoa
- 1 1/2 cups vegetable broth or water
- 1 tablespoon creamy peanut butter
- 3 tablespoons coconut milk
- 2 tablespoons sriracha sauce
- 2 tablespoons rice wine vinegar
- 1 tablespoon lime juice
- 1 teaspoon brown sugar
- 1/2 teaspoon garlic powder
- 1/2 teaspoon ground ginger
- 1 cup finely shredded carrots
- 1/2 cup chopped fresh cilantro leaves
- 2 scallions (thinly sliced)
- 2 tablespoons chopped salted roasted peanuts

Directions:
1. 1.Drain and rinse tofu, wrap in a clean dish towel or paper towels and place on a rimmed plate. Set another plate on top of wrapped tofu and weight top plate with something heavy to press out excess liquid. Let tofu stand for about 30 minutes
2. Cut tofu into bite-size cubes, toss with soy sauce and sesame oil to coat and season to taste with salt and pepper. Line a rimmed baking sheet with parchment paper. Spread tofu in a single layer on lined baking sheet and bake until crisp on all sides, about 45 minutes, turning about every 10 minutes.
3. Meanwhile, toast quinoa in a dry medium nonstick skillet over medium heat until golden brown, stirring occasionally, about 5 minutes. Add broth to quinoa and season to taste with salt and pepper. Reduce heat, cover skillet and simmer quinoa until liquid is absorbed and grain is tender, about 15 minutes. Fluff quinoa with a fork and set aside.
4. For the sauce, slightly melt peanut butter in the microwave for about 10 seconds. Whisk peanut butter, coconut milk, sriracha sauce, rice wine vinegar, lime juice, brown sugar, garlic powder and ground ginger until smooth. Season sauce to taste with salt and pepper and set aside.
5. Toss quinoa, tofu, carrots, cilantro and scallions to combine. Drizzle sauce over quinoa mixture and toss to coat. Scoop quinoa mixture into 4 deep bowls and sprinkle with peanuts to serve. Enjoy!

Nutrition:Per Serving: Calories: 232; Total Fat: 10g; Saturated Fat: 4g; Protein: 12g; Carbs: 27g; Fiber: 5g; Sugar: 4g

Sheet Pan Chicken Stir-fry

Servings: 6
Cooking Time: 30 Minutes
Ingredients:
- Stir fry sauce
- 2 - tbs brown sugar
- 2 - tbs oyster sauce
- 2 - tbs soy sauce
- 1 - tbs hoisin
- 1 ½ - lb. chicken breast cut into thin strips
- 5 - cups stir fry veggies

Directions:
6. Preheat broiler to 350 degrees
7. In a medium-sized bowl, combine pan fried food sauce and whisk all fixings together.
8. Coat chicken in sauce, and
9. Dump chicken on a sheet skillet, and include the veggies in.
10. Blend them together to cover the veggies, and ensure it is one, even, layer on the sheet dish.
11. Heat for 30 minutes until chicken is cooked through

Nutrition: Calories: 248kcal;carbs: 25g;protein: 29g;fat: 3g;sugar: 3g

Mexican Cauliflower "rice"

Servings: 4
Cooking Time: 5 Minutes
Ingredients:
- 1 teaspoon ground cumin
- 1 teaspoon chili powder
- 1/2 teaspoon paprika
- 1/2 teaspoon ancho chili powder
- 1/2 teaspoon garlic powder
- 1/2 teaspoon onion powder
- 1 medium head cauliflower (cored, cut into florets)
- 1 tablespoon vegetable oil
- 1 tablespoon water, plus more if necessary
- Salt, to taste
- 1 tablespoon guacamole

Directions:
1. In a small bowl, mix cumin, chili powder, paprika, ancho chili powder, garlic powder and onion powder and set aside.
2. Pulse cauliflower florets in a food processor until grainy. Do not over-process or cauliflower will be too soft.
3. Heat oil in a medium nonstick skillet over medium heat and sauté cauliflower until tender and lightly golden, 4 to 5 minutes, stirring frequently.
4. Remove cauliflower from heat, sprinkle with water and stir to coat. Sprinkle spice mixture over cauliflower and season to taste with salt. Stir cauliflower to coat with spices, adding more water if necessary.
5. Spoon cauliflower into bowls, garnish with guacamole and serve immediately. Enjoy!
Nutrition:Per Serving: Calories: 73; Total Fat: 4g; Saturated Fat: 3g; Protein: 3g; Carbs: 8g; Fiber: 4g; Sugar: 3g

Orange Arugula Salad With Smoked Turkey

Servings: 4
Cooking Time: 10-15 Minutes
Ingredients:
- 3 oz arugula, torn
- 4 oz lamb's lettuce, torn
- 4 oz lettuce, torn
- 8 oz smoked turkey breast, chopped into bite-sized pieces
- 2 large oranges, peeled, sliced
- For dressing:
- ¼ cup Greek yogurt
- 3 tbsp lemon juice
- 1 tsp apple cider vinegar
- ¼ cup olive oil

Directions:
1. Combine arugula, lamb's lettuce, and lettuce in a large colander. Wash thoroughly under cold running water and drain well. Tear into small pieces and set aside.
2. Now, combine vegetables in a large bowl. Add turkey breast and toss well. Then add sliced oranges and set aside.
3. Place Greek yogurt in a small bowl. Add lemon juice, apple cider, and olive oil. Whisk together until fully combined.
4. Drizzle over salad and serve.
Nutrition:Per Serving: Net carbs 16.4 g;Fiber 3.1 g;Fats 11 g;Fatsr 4 g;Calories 231

Saucy Garlic Broccoli

Servings: 4
Cooking Time: 15 Minutes
Ingredients:
- 2 stalks broccoli (cut into bite-size pieces)
- Salt and freshly ground black pepper, to taste
- 1 tablespoon olive oil
- 2 garlic cloves (minced)
- 1 tablespoon ginger (minced)
- 2 cups chicken stock
- 2 tablespoons soy sauce
- 1/2 teaspoon red pepper flakes
- 2 tablespoons cornstarch
- 1/4 cup chopped salted cashews

Directions:
1. Pour water into a large saucepan to a depth of about 2 inches. Set steamer basket in saucepan, place broccoli in basket and season to taste with salt and pepper. Cover pan and steam over medium heat until broccoli is soft, 8 to minutes.
2. Transfer broccoli to a serving dish, cover to keep warm and set aside. Empty cooking water from pan.
3. For the sauce, in the same pan, heat oil over medium heat and sauté garlic and ginger for about 1 minute. Add chicken broth, soy sauce and red pepper flakes to pan, season to taste with salt and pepper and heat to a simmer, stirring occasionally, about 10 minutes.
4. Dissolve cornstarch in about 1/cup cold water, whisk into sauce and cook until sauce is thickened, stirring constantly, about 2 minutes.
5. Pour sauce over broccoli and stir gently to coat. Sprinkle cashews over broccoli and serve immediately. Enjoy!
Nutrition:Per Serving: Calories: 141; Total Fat: 8g; Saturated Fat: 1g; Protein: 5g; Carbs: 15g; Fiber: 3g; Sugar: 2g

Turkey Fajitas Bowls

Servings: 4
Cooking Time: 20 Minutes
Ingredients:

- ½ lb. Turkey breast
- 2 tbsps. Olive oil
- 1 tbsp. Lemon juice
- 1 crushed garlic
- ¾ tsp. Chopped chili pepper
- ½ tsp. Dried oregano
- 1 sliced bell pepper
- 1 medium tomato
- ½ c. Shredded cheddar cheese
- 4 tostada bowls
- 4 tbsps. Salsa

Directions:
1.	Add oregano, chili pepper, garlic, lemon juice and bsp. Olive oil to a medium bowl. Whisk to combine.
2.	Add turkey then toss to coat. Allow to marinate for about 30 min.
3.	Set a skillet over medium heat with remaining oil. Add bell pepper and allow to cook for 2 minutes, stirring.
4.	Add turkey and cook for 3 more minutes. Add tomato, stir and remove from heat.
5.	Spoon mixture evenly into tostada bowls.
6.	Garnish with cheese and salsa then serve.
Nutrition: Calories: 240, fat: 15g, carbs: 5g, protein: 23g

Salmon Soba Noodle Miso Bowl Print

Servings: 1
Cooking Time: 15 Minutes
Ingredients:

- Salt
- 1 - ounce dried soba noodles
- 1 - tablespoon white miso paste
- 3 - cups of filtered water
- 2 - teaspoons mirin, optional
- 4 to 5 - cauliflower florets
- 3 - ounce filet of wild-caught salmon
- ½ - baby bok choy, ends trimmed
- Sesame seeds

Directions:
1.	Bring a medium pot of salted water, set over medium warmth, to a moderate bubble. Include the soba noodles and cook for around 4 to 5 minutes (the bundle consistently says like minutes and that is way excessively long, so give it a taste at the 4minutes imprint to ensure it's everything great). Expel when it's exceptionally still somewhat firm since we'll be cooking it again toward the end. Channel and put in a safe spot.
2.	In a similar void medium pot (no compelling reason to wash it out, excessively apathetic!) You cooked the soba noodles, include the miso glue and water. Turn the warmth to medium and give it a blend until the miso glue has broken down around 5 minutes. Include around 1/teaspoon of salt and mirin. Blend and give it a taste; modify the salt as indicated by taste. Turn the warmth to low and save.
3.	Preheat the broiler to 0 degrees f. Sprinkle the salmon on the two sides with a couple of portions of salt. Warmth the olive oil in a little sauté container set over medium-high heat. At the point

when the oil is flickering, include the cauliflower florets and cook for 2 to 3minutes. Expel and put in a safe spot. Include a teaspoon or two a greater amount of oil to the skillet. At the point when the oil was hot, include the salmon skin-side down; cook for 2 to 3minutes. Flip the salmon to the opposite side and move to the broiler to cook for an extra 5 minutes.
4.	In the interim, including the bok choy, saved soba noodles, and cauliflower to the miso blend, cook for an extra 2minutes until the bok choy turns somewhat delicate and the shading goes splendid green. Spoon into a bowl and top with the salmon.
Nutrition: Calories: 4;carbs: 36g;fat: 20g;protein: 32g

Savory Oatmeal With Cheddar And Fried Egg

Servings:1
Cooking Time: 8 Minutes
Ingredients:

- ¼- cup dry quick-cooking steel-cut oats
- ¾ - cup water
- Salt and pepper
- 2 - tablespoons shredded white cheddar cheese
- ¼ - cup diced red pepper
- 1 - large egg
- 2 - tablespoons finely chopped onions
- Chopped walnuts
- Optional toppings
- 1 - tsp coconut oil, divided
- Spice blend
- Sliced green onions

Directions:
1.	Bring water to bubble. Include oats, diminish the warmth a little and let it cook for about 3minutes until all fluid is assimilated. Mood killer warmth and mix in cheddar, a little squeeze of salt, and pepper.
2.	Warm a nonstick dish with ½ teaspoon of coconut oil over medium-high heat. Include vegetables and cook for to 3minutes, until they mollify. Spoon vegetables over cooked oats. Diminish warmth to medium.
3.	Include staying ½ teaspoon of oil and fry an egg. Cook until the whites are never again translucent and serve over oats.
4.	Top with slashed pecans, green onions, and za'atar, on the off chance that you like.
Nutrition: Calories: 307;carbs: 31g;fat: 1;protein: 14g

Cheesy Cauliflower Casserole

Servings: 3
Cooking Time: 20 Minutes
Ingredients:
- 1 small head cauliflower (about 12 ounces, cut into bite-size pieces)
- 1/2 cup plain unsweetened nonfat yogurt
- 1 package (3 ounces) cream cheese (cut into small cubes)
- 1/2 teaspoon garlic salt
- 1/4 teaspoon onion powder
- Dash of red pepper flakes, to taste
- Salt and freshly ground black pepper, to taste
- Nonstick cooking spray
- 1/4 cup (about 1 ounce) shredded cheddar cheese

Directions:
1. Preheat oven to 350°F.
2. Steam cauliflower just until softened, about 5 minutes. Add yogurt, cream cheese, garlic salt, onion powder and red pepper flakes to cauliflower, season to taste with salt and pepper and toss gently to coat
3. Spray a small glass casserole dish with nonstick cooking spray. Evenly spread cauliflower mixture in casserole dish and sprinkle with cheddar cheese.
4. Bake casserole until cheese is melted, about 15 minutes. Serve immediately and enjoy!
Nutrition:Per Serving: Calories: 181; Total Fat: 13g; Saturated Fat: 8g; Protein: 8g; Carbs: 9g; Fiber: 2g; Sugar:

Healthy Sheet Pan Chicken Fajitas

Servings: 6
Cooking Time: 20 Minutes
Ingredients:
- 3 - boneless skinless chicken breasts pounded
- 4 - bell peppers, sliced any color
- 1 - large onion, sliced
- 4 - tablespoons olive oil divided
- Salt and pepper to taste
- 1 - teaspoon garlic powder
- 1 - teaspoon chili powder
- 1 - teaspoon cumin
- ½ - teaspoon cayenne pepper
- Juice of 1 lime
- 8 6 - inch flour tortillas
- Toppings:
- Light sour cream
- Salsa
- Mashed
- Chopped cilantro
- Lime wedges for squeezing

Directions:
1. Preheat stove to 375 degrees and daintily oil a huge sheet skillet. Mix together garlic powder, stew powder, cumin, and cayenne pepper.
2. Organize chicken bosoms on the container, shower with tablespoons olive oil and rub in with your fingers on the two sides. Season liberally with salt on the two sides, at that point season chicken with blended flavors on the two sides.
3. Organize cut peppers and onions on the container around the chicken bosoms. Shower with staying 2 tablespoons olive oil. Season liberally with salt.
4. Prepare for 15 to 20 minutes until chicken is cooked through. Move chicken to a cutting board, return peppers and onions to the stove and change to broil for 3 to 5 minutes until the edges of the veggies begin to singe marginally, at that point expel from broiler.
5. While veggies are searing, shower new lime squeeze over chicken at that point daintily cut into strips.
6. Gather fajitas with chicken, peppers, onions, and wanted garnishes and serve right away.
Nutrition: Calories: 241;carbs: ;fat: 16g;protein: 17g

Tandoori Chicken

Servings: 6
Cooking Time: 35 Minutes
Ingredients:
- 1 c. Plain yogurt
- ½ c, lemon juice
- 5 crushed garlic cloves
- 2 tbsps. Paprika
- 1 tsp. Yellow curry powder
- 1 tsp. Ground ginger
- 6 skinless chicken breasts
- 6 skewers

Directions:
1. Set oven to 400 degrees f. In blender, combine red pepper flakes, ginger, curry, paprika, garlic, lemon juice and yogurt, then process into a smooth paste.
2. Add chicken strips evenly onto skewers. Add chicken to a shallow casserole dish then cover with ½ of yogurt mixture.
3. Tightly seal and rest in refrigerator for about 15 minutes.
4. Lightly grease a baking tray, then transfer chicken skewers onto it, and top with remaining yogurt mixture.
5. Set to bake until the chicken is fully cooked. Serve and enjoy.
Nutrition: Calories: 177, fat: 7.2g, carbs: , protein: 20.6g

Veggie Quesadillas With Cilantro Yogurt Dip

Servings: 3
Cooking Time: 25 Minutes
Ingredients:
- 1 c. Black beans
- 2 tbsps. Chopped cilantro
- ½ chopped bell pepper
- ½ c. Corn kernels
- 1 c. Shredded cheese
- 6 corn tortillas
- 1 shredded carrot

Directions:
1.   Set skillet to preheat on low heat. Lay 3 tortillas on a flat surface.
2.   Top evenly with peppers, carrots, cilantro, beans, corn and cheese over the tortillas, covering each with another tortilla, maximum.
3.   Add quesadilla to preheated skillet. Cook until the cheese melts and tortilla is a nice golden brown (about 2 min).
4.   Flip quesadilla and cook for about a minute or until golden.
5.   Mix well. Slice each quesadilla into 4 even wedges and serve with dip. Enjoy!
Nutrition: Calories: 344, fat: 8g, carbs: 4, protein: 27g

Healthy Pita Pizza With Goat Cheese

Servings:1
Cooking Time: 10 Minutes
Ingredients:
- 4 - whole-wheat pitas
- 1 - small red onion
- Handful thyme sprigs
- 1 - pound tomatoes
- 2 - cups shredded mozzarella cheese
- 4 - ounces goat cheese
- Kosher salt
- Fresh ground pepper
- Olive oil (optional)

Directions:
1.   Spot a pizza stone in the broiler and preheat to 450°f.
2.   Spot pita straightforwardly on the stove grind and pre-heat 3 minutes for each side, at that point flip and prepare an additional 3 minutes.
3.   In the interim, daintily cut the red onion. Generally, hack the thyme. Utilizing a serrated blade, meagerly cut the tomatoes.
4.   At the point when the pitas are fresh, expel them from the stove. The top each with 1/2 cup mozzarella, at that point tomatoes, onions, and thyme leaves. Include dabs of goat cheddar.
5.   Sprinkle generously with fit salt, particularly the tomatoes. Whenever wanted, shower with olive oil. Heat until the cheddar is softened, around minutes. Take out from the broiler, cut into wedges, and serve.

Nutrition: Calories: 283;carbs: 40g;fat: 9g;protein: 12g

Baked Dijon Salmon

Servings: 6
Cooking Time: 10 Minutes
Ingredients:
- 1 lb salmon
- 3 tbsp olive oil
- 1 tsp ginger, grated
- 2 tbsp Dijon mustard
- 1 tsp pepper
- Salt

Directions:
1.   In a small bowl, mix together oil, mustard, ginger, and pepper.
2.   Preheat the oven to 400 F/ 0 C.
3.   Spray a baking tray with cooking spray and set aside.
4.   Place salmon on a baking tray and spread oil mixture over salmon evenly.
5.   Bake salmon for 10 minutes.
6.   Serve and enjoy.
Nutrition:Per Servings: Calories 165 Fat 11.9 g Carbohydrates 0.g Sugar 0.1 g Protein 15 g Cholesterol 33 mg

Grilled Chicken Breasts

Servings: 4
Cooking Time: 15 Minutes
Ingredients:
- 2 lbs chicken breasts, halves
- 6 tbsp fresh parsley, minced
- 6 tbsp olive oil
- 1 1/2 tsp dried oregano
- 1 tsp paprika
- 1 tbsp garlic, minced
- 6 tbsp fresh lemon juice
- Pepper
- Salt

Directions:
1.   Pierce chicken breasts using a fork. Season with pepper and salt.
2.   Add lemon juice, oregano, paprika, garlic, parsley, and olive oil into the zip-lock bag.
3.   Add chicken to the zip-lock bag.
4.   Seal bag and shake well and place in the refrigerator for 1-2 hours.
5.   Heat grill over medium-high heat.
6.   Place marinated chicken on the grill and cook for 5-minutes on each side.
7.   Serve and enjoy.
Nutrition:Per Servings: Calories 625 Fat 3g Carbohydrates 2 g Sugar 0.6 g Protein 65 g Cholesterol 200 mg

Mediterranean Tuna Salad

Servings: 4
Cooking Time: 30 Minutes
Ingredients:
- 1 small red onion (julienned)
- 1/4 cup vinegar
- 2 cans or jars (about 6 ounces each) Ventresca tuna (drained)
- 1 celery stalk (cut into thin 1" pieces)
- 1/4 cup pitted black olives (cut into strips)
- 1/4 cup chopped parsley leaves
- 1 tablespoon capers (halved if necessary)
- 1/4 cup extra-virgin olive oil
- 1 teaspoon lemon juice
- 1 teaspoon Worcestershire sauce
- 1 teaspoon fish sauce
- Salt and freshly ground black pepper, to taste

Directions:
1. Mix onion and vinegar and let stand for about minutes.
2. In a large bowl, flake tuna into large chunks. Add celery, olives, parsley and capers and toss gently to combine.
3. Mix olive oil, lemon juice, Worcestershire sauce and fish sauce, drizzle over tuna mixture and toss gently to combine.
4. Drain onions and discard vinegar. Add onions to tuna mixture, season to taste with salt and pepper and toss gently to combine. Serve tuna salad immediately, or refrigerate until chilled through before serving. Enjoy!

Nutrition:Per Serving: Calories: 244; Total Fat: 18g; Saturated Fat: 2g; Protein: 14g; Carbs: ; Fiber: 2g; Sugar: 1g

Skillet Salmon With Tomato Quinoa

Servings:1
Cooking Time: 15 Minutes
Ingredients:
- 2 - teaspoons canola oil
- 3 - cloves garlic, finely chopped
- 1 - cup cooked quinoa
- ¾ - cup canned diced tomatoes
- ¼ - teaspoon paprika
- Salt
- Pepper
- 1 - cup loosely packed baby spinach
- 2 - tablespoons fresh basil, chopped
- 1 - salmon filet

Directions:
1. Warm stove to 425°.
2. In a little ovenproof skillet over medium warmth, heat oil. Include garlic and cook, mixing, until fragrant, around 1 moment. Include quinoa, tomatoes, and paprika. Season with salt and pepper. Cook, mixing until warmed through. Include spinach and basil and blend to wither.
3. Season salmon generously with salt and pepper. Spot salmon over the quinoa blend. Move to broiler and meal 8 to 12minutes for medium-uncommon, 12 to 18minutes for all-around done.
4. Give scraps a chance to cool totally before putting away in a water/air proof compartment in the refrigerator.

Nutrition: Calories: 3;fat 18g;carbs 54g;sugar 6g;protein 30g

Sweet Potatoes With Egg Whites

Servings: 4
Cooking Time: 35-40 Minutes
Ingredients:
- 4 medium sweet potatoes, peeled6 large eggs
- 2 medium onions, peeled
- 1 tbsp ground garlic
- 4 tbsp olive oil
- ½ tsp sea salt
- ¼ tsp ground pepper

Directions:
1. Preheat your oven to 350 degrees.
2. Spread tablespoons of olive oil over a medium sized baking sheet. Place the potatoes on the baking sheet. Bake for about 20 minutes.
3. Remove from the oven and allow it to cool for a while. Lower the oven heat to 200 degrees.
4. Meanwhile, chop the onions into small pieces. Separate egg whites from yolks. Cut the potatoes into thick slices and place them in a bowl.
5. Add chopped onions, 2 tablespoons of olive oil, egg whites, ground garlic, sea salt and pepper. Mix well.
6. Spread this mixture over a baking sheet and bake for another 15-20 minutes.

Nutrition:Per Serving: Net carbs 14.2 g;Fiber 2 g;Fats 21.6 g;Fatsr 2 g;Calories 285

Spinach Shrimp Alfredo

Servings: 2
Cooking Time: 15 Minutes
Ingredients:
- 1/2 lb. Shrimp, deveined
- 2 garlic cloves, minced
- 2 tbsp onion, chopped
- 1 cup fresh spinach, chopped
- 1/2 cup heavy cream
- 1 tbsp butter
- Pepper
- Salt

Directions:
1. Melt butter in a pan over medium heat.
2. Add onion, garlic and shrimp in the pan and sauté for 3 minutes.
3. Add remaining ingredients and simmer for 7 minutes or until cooked.
4. Serve and enjoy.

Nutrition: Calories 300;Fat 19 g;Carbohydrates g;Sugar 0.5 g;Protein 27 g;Cholesterol 295 mg

Grilled Veal Steak With Vegetables

Servings: 4
Cooking Time: 35 Minutes
Ingredients:
- 1 lb. veal steak, about 1 inch thick
- 1 medium red pepper
- 1 medium green pepper
- 1 small onion, finely chopped
- 3 tbsp olive oil
- Salt and pepper to taste

Directions:
1. Wash and pat dry the steak with kitchen paper. Heat up the olive oil over medium temperature in a non-stick grill pan and fry for about 20 minutes (about on each side). Remove from the heat and set aside.
2. Wash and cut vegetables into thin strips. Add some salt and pepper. Add to a grill pan and cook for about 15 minutes, stirring constantly.
3. Serve immediately.

Nutrition:Per Serving: Net carbs 5.3 g; Fiber 1.3 g; Fats 18.5 g; Fatsr 2 g; Calories 311

Broiled Fish Fillet

Servings: 2
Cooking Time: 10 Minutes
Ingredients:
- 2 cod fish fillets
- 1/8 tsp curry powder
- 2 tsp butter
- 1/4 tsp paprika
- 1/8 tsp pepper
- 1/8 tsp salt

Directions:
1. Preheat the broiler.
2. Spray broiler pan with cooking spray and set aside.
3. In a small bowl, mix together paprika, curry powder, pepper, and salt.
4. Coat fish fillet with paprika mixture and place on broiler pan.
5. Broil fish for 10-12 minutes.
6. Top with butter and serve.

Nutrition:Per Servings: Calories 224 Fat 5.4 g Carbohydrates 0.3 g Sugar 0 g Protein 41.2 g Cholesterol 109 mg

Spaghetti Squash Lasagna V

Servings: 6
Cooking Time: 1-hour 50 Minutes
Ingredients:
- 2 c. Marinara sauce
- 3 c. Roasted spaghetti squash
- 1 c. Ricotta
- 8 tsps. Grated parmesan cheese
- 6 oz. Shredded mozzarella cheese
- 1/4 tsp. Red pepper flakes

Directions:
1. Set oven to preheat oven to 375 degrees f and spoon half of marinara sauce into baking dish.
2. Top with squash, then layer remaining ingredients.
3. Cover and set to bake until cheese are melted and edges brown (about 20 minutes).
4. Remove cover and return to bake for another 5 minutes. Enjoy!

Nutrition: Calories: 2, fat: 15.9g, carbs: 5.5g, protein: 21.4g

Roasted Kielbasa And Cabbage

Servings: 4
Cooking Time: 35 Minutes
Ingredients:
- Mustard vinaigrette
- 1/4 - cup olive oil
- 2 - tbsp red wine vinegar
- 1 - tbsp stone ground or whole grain mustard
- 1 - small clove garlic, crushed or minced
- 1/4 - tsp salt
- Freshly cracked pepper
- Roasted kielbasa and vegetables
- 1/2 - lb. kielbasa
- 1 - lb. baby red potatoes
- 1/2 - head cabbage
- 2 - tbsp olive oil, divided
- Pinch of salt and pepper
- Handful chopped fresh parsley

Directions:
1. Preheat the broiler to 400ºf. In a bit bowl whisk collectively the olive oil, red wine vinegar, mustard, squashed garlic, salt, and crisply cut up pepper for the vinaigrette. Put the French dressing in a secure spot.
2. Cut the kielbasa into 1/4 inch thick. Wash the potatoes properly and cut them into 1/4 inch adjusts also. Set the kielbasa and potatoes on a big heating sheet and sprinkle with 1 tbsp olive oil. Toss the kielbasa and potatoes in the oil till they're all around included and the outside of the heating sheet is likewise canvassed in oil. Sprinkle a touch of salt and pepper over top.
3. Take any dirty or harmed leaves out from the cabbage. Cut the stem off the cabbage, at that factor reduce it down the center. Hold one half for an alternate formulation. Cut the staying half into 1-inch extensive cuts. Cut every cut into portions. Spot the cabbage portions on the heating sheet with the kielbasa and potatoes, settling them down so they are laying level at the getting ready sheet.
4. Brush the staying 1 tbsp olive oil over the outdoor of the cabbage pieces and consist of the closing squeeze of salt and pepper to each.
5. Cook the kielbasa, potatoes, and cabbage within the preheated broiler for 20mins. Take the heating sheet out from the range and carefully turn the kielbasa, potatoes, and cabbage pieces. The cabbage may additionally self-destruct a chunk as it's flipped, that's o.k. Return the heating sheet to the broiler and dish for an extra 10-1minutes, or until the cabbage is sensitive and the rims are particularly darkish-colored and fresh. The kielbasa and potato cuts need to be all-around seared.
6. Take the preparing sheet out from the broiler and top with new slashed parsley and a sprinkle of the mustard vinaigrette. Servings heat.

Nutrition: Calories: 269; carbs: 19g; fat: 13g; protein: 22g

48

Delicious Minced Pork

Servings: 3
Cooking Time: 20 Minutes
Ingredients:
- 14 oz minced pork
- 1/4 cup green bell pepper, chopped
- 1/2 onion, chopped
- 2 tbsp water
- ¼ tsp cumin powder
- 3/4 cup ketchup, sugar-free
- 1/2 tbsp olive oil
- Pepper
- Salt

Directions:
1. Heat oil in pan over medium heat.
2. Add pepper and onion and sauté until soften.
3. Add meat, pepper, cumin powder, and salt and cook until browned.
4. Add water and ketchup and stir well. Bring to boil.
5. Serve and enjoy.
Nutrition: Calories 275;Fat 7 g;Carbohydrates 14 g;Sugar 13 g;Protein 3g;Cholesterol 95 mg

Cinnamon Olive Pork Chops

Servings: 6
Cooking Time: 30 Minutes
Ingredients:
- 6 pork chops, boneless and cut into thick slices
- 1/2 cup olives, pitted and sliced
- 7.5 oz ragu
- 1 tbsp olive oil
- 1/4 cup beef broth
- 3 garlic cloves, chopped
- 1/8 tsp ground cinnamon
- 1 large onion, sliced

Directions:
1. Heat oil in a pan over medium-high heat.
2. Add pork chops in a pan and cook until lightly brown and set aside.
3. Cook garlic and onion and cook until onion is softened.
4. Add broth and bring to boil.
5. Return pork chops to pan and stir in ragu and remaining ingredients.
6. Cover and simmer for 20 minutes.
7. Serve and enjoy.
Nutrition: Calories 320;Fat 22 g;Carbohydrates 6 g;Sugar 1 g;Protein 20 g;Cholesterol 70 mg

Honey Garlic Chicken Sheet Pan Dinner

Servings: 4
Cooking Time: 35 To 40 Minutes
Ingredients:
- ¼ - cup chicken broth or water
- 1/3 - cup honey
- 6 - cloves garlic, minced
- 2 - tbsp rice wine vinegar
- 1 - tbsp soy sauce
- 2 - tsp garlic powder
- Salt and pepper, to taste
- 2 - large potatoes, washed and chopped into 1″ pieces
- 5 to 6 - chicken legs
- 1 - broccoli crown, chopped

Directions:
1. Preheat broiler to 425 f. What's more, oil a sheet dish.
2. Join the chicken soup, nectar, minced garlic, rice wine vinegar, soy sauce, and garlic powder in a blending bowl. Add hacked potatoes to the bowl and blend to cover well. Spoon potatoes onto the readied heating sheet utilizing an opened spoon so as to hold fluid in the blending bowl.
3. Add chicken legs to the rest of the sauce in the bowl and coat well. Spot the covered chicken over the potatoes and pour remaining sauce over chicken legs in the skillet. Season chicken legs with salt and pepper.
4. Add hacked broccoli to the sheet skillet.
5. Prepare for 3to 40minutes or until chicken is never again pink and squeezes run clear.
6. Servings honey garlic chicken sheet pan dinner, as a simple one-dish supper!
Nutrition: Calories: 23carbs: 5g;fat: 11g;protein: 27g

Breakfast Almond Freezer Pops

Servings: 8
Cooking Time: 10 Minutes Plus 4 Hours Freezing
Ingredients:
- 2 cups plain unsweetened Greek yogurt
- 1 cup almond milk
- 2 ripe bananas (mashed)
- 1/4 cup almond butter
- 1 cup chopped strawberries

Directions:
1. Whisk yogurt, milk and bananas until smooth. Add strawberries and almonds and stir until combined.
2. Spoon yogurt mixture into 6 freezer pop molds, set handled lids in place and freeze until firm, about 4 hours. Pops will keep in the freezer for about weeks. Serve as desired and enjoy!
Nutrition:Per Serving: Calories: 1; Total Fat: 9g; Saturated Fat: 7g; Protein: 4g; Carbs: 11g; Fiber: 2g; Sugar: 7g

Flavorful Pork Chops

Servings: 4
Cooking Time: 8 Hours
Ingredients:
- 4 pork chops, boneless
- 1/2 tbsp garlic powder
- 1 tbsp paprika
- 3 garlic cloves, minced
- 1 cup vegetable broth
- 1/4 cup olive oil
- 1/2 tsp dried basil
- 1/2 tsp dried oregano
- 1 tbsp Italian seasoning
- Pepper
- Salt

Directions:
1. In a bowl, whisk together basil, oregano, Italian seasoning, garlic powder, paprika, garlic, broth, and olive oil. Pour into the crock pot.
2. Season pork chops with pepper and salt and place into the crock pot.
3. Cover and cook on low for 8 hours.
4. Serve and enjoy.
Nutrition: Calories 390;Fat 32 g;Carbohydrates 4 g;Sugar 1 g;Protein 20 g;Cholesterol 70 mg

Garlic Shrimp

Servings: 4
Cooking Time: 15 Minutes
Ingredients:
- 1 lb. Shrimp, peeled and deveined
- 1 tsp parsley, chopped
- 2 tbsp lemon juice
- 5 garlic cloves, minced
- 3 tbsp butter
- Salt

Directions:
1. Melt butter in a pan over high heat.
2. Add shrimp in pan and cook for 1 minutes. Season with salt.
3. Stir and cook shrimp until turn to pink.
4. Add lemon juice and garlic and cook for 2 minutes.
5. Turn heat to medium and cook for 4 minutes more.
6. Garnish with parsley and serve.
Nutrition: Calories 219;Fat 10.6 g;Carbohydrates 3.2 g;Sugar 0.2 g;Protein 26 g;Cholesterol 262 mg

Coconut Flour Spinach Casserole

Servings: 6
Cooking Time: 1 Hour
Ingredients:
- 4 eggs
- ¾ c. Unsweetened almond milk
- 3 oz. Chopped spinach
- 3 oz. Chopped artichoke hearts
- 1 c. Grated parmesan
- 3 minced garlic cloves
- 1 tsp. Salt
- ½ tsp. Pepper
- ¾ c. Coconut flour
- 1 tbsp. Baking powder

Directions:
1. Preheat air fryer to 375 degrees f. Grease air fryer pan with cooking spray.
2. Whisk eggs with almond milk, spinach, artichoke hearts and ½ cup of parmesan cheese. Add salt, garlic and pepper.
3. Add the coconut flour and baking powder; whisk until well combined.
4. Spread mixture into air fryer pan and sprinkle remaining cheese over it.
5. Place the baking pan in the air fryer and cook for about 30 minutes.
6. Remove baking pan from air fryer and sprinkle with chopped basil. Slice, then serve and enjoy!
Nutrition: Calories: 1.2, fat: 10.3g, carbs: 2.4g, protein: 17.7g

Loaded Sweet Potatoes

Servings: 4
Cooking Time: 35 Minutes
Ingredients:
- 4 medium sweet potatoes, baked
- ½ c. Greek yogurt
- 1 tsp. Taco seasoning
- 1 tsp. Olive oil
- 1 diced red pepper
- ½ diced red onion
- 1 1/3 c. Canned black beans
- ½ c. Mexican cheese blend
- ¼ c. Chopped cilantro
- ½ c. Salsa

Directions:
1. Mix taco seasoning and yogurt well, then set aside.
2. Set a skillet over medium heat with oil to get hot.
3. Add in remaining ingredients, except potatoes, cheese and salsa, and cook for about 8 minutes or until fully heated through.
4. Slightly pierce potatoes down the center and top evenly with all remaining ingredients. Serve.
Nutrition: Calories: 311, fat: 8.3g, carbs: g, protein: 3.2g

Cheesy Bell Pepper Scramble

Servings: 2
Cooking Time: 10 Minutes
Ingredients:
- 1 tablespoon butter
- 1/4 cup diced red bell pepper
- 1/4 cup diced green bell pepper
- 1/4 cup diced onion
- 1 garlic clove (minced)
- 4 eggs (lightly beaten)
- 2 tablespoons skim milk
- Salt and freshly ground black pepper, to taste
- 2 tablespoons grated mild cheddar cheese

Directions:
1. Melt butter in a medium nonstick skillet over medium heat and sauté bell peppers and onions until soft, about 5 minutes, stirring occasionally. Add garlic and sauté about minute more, stirring constantly.
2. Whisk eggs and milk until thoroughly combined, add to bell pepper mixture and season to taste with salt and pepper. Cook and stir until eggs are completely set and cooked through, 5 to 6 minutes.
3. Season eggs to taste with salt and pepper, sprinkle with cheese and serve immediately. Enjoy!
Nutrition:Per Serving: Calories: 228; Total Fat: 17g; Saturated Fat: 8g; Protein: 1; Carbs: 6g; Fiber: 1g; Sugar: 4g

Sweet Roasted Beet & Arugula Tortilla Pizza V

Servings: 6
Cooking Time: 25 Minutes
Ingredients:
- 2 chopped beets
- 6 corn tortillas
- 1 c. Arugula
- ½ c. Goat cheese
- 1 c. Blackberries
- 2 tbsps. Honey
- 2 tbsps. Balsamic vinegar

Directions:
1. Preheat oven to 350 f. Lay tortillas on a flat surface.
2. Top with beets, berries and goat cheese. Combine balsamic vinegar and honey together in a small bowl, and whisk to combine.
3. Drizzle the mixture over pizza and to bake for about 10 minutes, or until cheese has melted slightly and tortilla is crisp.
4. Garnish with arugula and serve.
Nutrition: Calories: 286, fat: 40g, carbs: 42g, protein: 1

Zoodles With Pesto

Servings: 4
Cooking Time: 10 Minutes
Ingredients:
- 3 medium zucchini (about 12 ounces total)
- 1 teaspoon salt, plus more to taste
- 2 tablespoons pine nuts
- 1/2 cup fresh basil leaves (stems removed)
- 1 garlic clove (minced)
- 1/2 teaspoon lemon juice
- 2 tablespoons extra virgin olive oil
- 2 tablespoons grated Romano cheese
- 1 tablespoon vegetable oil

Directions:
1. Cut zucchini into thin, noodle-like strips with a spiralizer, mandoline or vegetable peeler. Place zucchini in a colander, sprinkle with 2 teaspoon salt to draw out moisture and let stand while you prepare the pesto.
2. For the pesto, toast pine nuts in a medium dry nonstick skillet over medium heat until lightly browned, to 3 minutes, stirring frequently.
3. Process toasted pine nuts, basil, garlic, lemon juice and 1/4 teaspoon salt in a food processor and process until finely minced.
4. Continue processing pesto mixture, add olive oil in a slow thin stream and process until smooth. Add cheese and process just until combined.
5. Blot zoodles as dry as possible with paper towels. Heat vegetable oil in a medium nonstick skillet over medium heat and sauté zoodles until golden, 3 to 4 minutes, stirring frequently. Season zoodles with remaining 1/4 teaspoon salt plus more to taste.
6. Spoon zoodles onto 4 plates, top with pesto and serve immediately. Enjoy!
Nutrition:Per Serving: Calories: 161; Total Fat: 16g; Saturated Fat: 5g; Protein: 4g; Carbs: 1g; Fiber: 1g; Sugar: 0g

Dijon Potato Salad

Servings: 5
Cooking Time: 20 Minutes
Ingredients:
- 1 lb. potatoes
- 1/2 lime juice
- 2 tbsp olive oil
- 2 tbsp fresh dill, chopped
- 2 tbsp chives, minced
- 1/2 tbsp vinegar
- 1 tbsp Dijon mustard
- 1/2 lime zest
- Pepper
- Salt

Directions:
1. Add water in a large pot and bring to boil.
2. Add potatoes in boiling water and cook for 15 minutes or until tender. Drain well and set aside.
3. In a small bowl, whisk together vinegar, mustard, lime zest, lime juice, olive oil, dill, and chives.
4. Peel potatoes and diced and transfer in mixing bowl.
5. Pour vinegar mixture over potatoes and stir to coat.
6. Season with pepper and salt.
7. Serve and enjoy.
Nutrition: Calories 115;Fat 6 g;Carbohydrates 15 g;Sugar 1 g;Protein 2 g;Cholesterol 0 mg

Sheet Pan Cauliflower Nachos

Servings: 6
Cooking Time: 20 Minutes
Ingredients:
- 1 - head cauliflower, cut into florets
- 2 - t-spoon olive oil
- ¼ - t-spoon chili powder
- 3 - cloves garlic, minced
- ½ - t-spoon cumin
- ¼ - teaspoon smoked paprika
- Kosher salt and freshly ground black pepper,
- 6 - ounces tortilla chips
- 1 - (15-ounce) can black beans, drained and rinsed
- 1 - cup shredded cheddar cheese
- 1 - roma tomato, diced
- 1/3 - cup guacamole, homemade
- ¼ - cup diced red onion
- 1 - jalapeno, thinly sliced
- 2 - t-spoon chopped fresh cilantro leaves

Directions:
1. Preheat stove to 425 degrees f. Softly oil a heating sheet.
2. Spot cauliflower florets in a solitary layer onto the readied heating sheet. Include olive oil, garlic, cumin, bean stew powder, and paprika; season with salt and pepper, to taste. Tenderly hurl to consolidate. Spot into the stove and prepare for 1 to 14 minutes, or until delicate and brilliant darker.
3. Blend in tortilla contributes a solitary layer. Top with dark beans and cheddar.
4. Spot into the stove and prepare until warmed through and the cheddar liquefies around 5 to 6 minutes.
5. Servings promptly; beat with tomato, guacamole, onion, jalapeno, and cilantro.

Nutrition: Calories: 404;carbs: 5g;fat: 23g;protein: 42g

Crunchy Tuna Salad

Servings: 4
Cooking Time: 20 Minutes
Ingredients:
- 1/2 cup low-fat cottage cheese
- 1/2 cup plain unsweetened yogurt
- 2 tablespoons diced yellow or orange bell pepper
- 2 tablespoons diced red onion
- 1 tablespoon chopped parsley leaves
- 2 cans (5 ounces each) tuna in water (well drained)
- 2 ounces mild cheddar cheese (cut into 1/4" cubes)

Directions:
1. Mash cottage cheese with a fork to break up larger curds. Add yogurt, bell pepper, onion and parsley and mix well.
2. Crumble tuna with a fork and add to cottage cheese mixture with cheese cubes. Mix gently until combined. Serve as desired and enjoy!

Nutrition:Per Serving: Calories: 21 Total Fat: 8g; Saturated Fat: 4g; Protein: 29g; Carbs: 7g; Fiber: 1g; Sugar: 4g

Shrimp Scampi For One

Servings: 1
Cooking Time: 15 Minutes
Ingredients:
- ¼ - pound 21 count shrimp, about 6
- 1 - large shallot, minced
- 2 to 3 - cloves garlic, minced
- 2 - tablespoons butter
- 3 - tablespoons cream
- Splash of white wine (optional)
- 1/8 - teaspoon crushed red pepper flakes (optional)
- Parmesan cheese (optional)
- Salt and pepper
- Spaghetti
- ¼ - cup reserved pasta water

Directions:
1. Cook pasta as indicated by the bundle. Hold a portion of the cooking water for the sauce later. Channel the pasta and put it in a safe spot.
2. Mince garlic and shallots and clean the shrimp in the event that they aren't as of now cleaned.
3. Add spread to pot over medium warmth. When hot and liquefied, include the cleaned shrimp and cook for 90 seconds for every side. At that point include shallots and garlic and cook for an additional seconds until delicate.
4. Include a sprinkle of white wine and the squashed red pepper. Do whatever it takes not to overcook them.
5. Add cream to the shrimp and blend. The sauce ought to decrease pleasantly.
6. Include pasta over into the pot and blend to join. Season with salt and pepper. On the off chance that the sauce is excessively thick, include a touch of saved pasta water to thin it out. Try not to make it excessively slim, however!

Nutrition: Calories: 835;fat 43.5g;carbs 62.2g;sugars 2.4g;protein 45.5g

Sheet Pan Sweet And Sour Chicken

Servings: 6
Cooking Time: 40 Minutes
Ingredients:
- 1 - large onion
- 2 - green bell peppers
- 1 - red bell pepper
- 20 - oz can pineapple chunks
- 2 - boneless skinless chicken breasts (about 1.25 lb.)
- 2 - tbsp cooking oil
- ¼ - tsp garlic powder
- ½ - tsp ground ginger
- Salt and pepper to taste
- ¼ - cup ketchup
- ¼ - cup brown sugar
- 1/3 - cup rice or apple cider vinegar
- 1.5 - tbsp soy sauce
- 1.5 - tbsp cornstarch
- 3 - green onions, sliced
- 6 - cups cooked rice

Directions:
1. Preheat the broiler to 400°f. Cut the onion, ringer peppers, and chicken bosoms into one-inch pieces. Channel the pineapple well, holding the juice for the sauce. Spot the onion, chime pepper, chicken, and pineapple lumps on an enormous sheet container in a solitary layer. Utilize two sheets, if necessary, to keep the chicken and vegetables from heaping over one another. They need a little space to darker effectively.
2. Sprinkle the cooking oil over the fixings on the sheet skillet, trailed by the garlic powder, ground ginger, and a squeeze or two of salt and pepper. Hurl the chicken, chime peppers, onions, and pineapple until they are equitably covered in oil and flavors.
3. Heat the chicken and vegetables in the broiler for about 40minutes, or until they are somewhat cooked on the edges. Blend part of the way through the preparing time to redistribute the warmth and enable abundance dampness to dissipate.
4. While the chicken and vegetables are heating, set up the sauce. In a little saucepot whisk together the held pineapple juice (around 1 cup), ketchup, dark colored sugar, vinegar, soy sauce, and cornstarch until the cornstarch is completely broken down. Warmth the blend over medium fire, mixing regularly, until it starts to stew. When it starts to stew the cornstarch will start to gel and thicken the sauce. When the sauce has thickened to a coating, expel it from the warmth and put it aside until prepared to utilize.
5. At the point when the chicken and vegetables have got done with heating, take them out from the stove and pour the readied sauce over top. Blend until everything is covered in sauce.
6. Servings the sweet and harsh chicken over cooked rice with cut green onions sprinkled over top.

Nutrition: Calories: 290;carbs: 54g;fat: 5g;protein: 8g

Simple Grilled Pork Tenderloin

Servings: 8
Cooking Time: 30 Minutes
Ingredients:
- 2 lbs. Pork tenderloin
- 2 tbsp ranch dressing mix
- 2 tbsp olive oil

Directions:
1. Preheat the grill to 350 f.
2. Brush pork loin with oil and season with ranch dressing.
3. Place pork loin on hot grill and cook for minutes. Turn tenderloin every 10 minutes.
4. Slice and serve.

Nutrition: Calories 17Fat 7 g;Carbohydrates 2 g;Sugar 2 g;Protein 23 g;Cholesterol 73 mg

Pork Egg Roll Bowl

Servings: 6
Cooking Time: 10 Minutes
Ingredients:
- 1 lb. Ground pork
- 3 tbsp soy sauce
- 1 tbsp sesame oil
- 1/2 onion, sliced
- 1 medium cabbage head, sliced
- 2 tbsp green onion, chopped
- 2 tbsp chicken broth
- 1 tsp ground ginger
- 2 garlic cloves, minced
- Pepper
- Salt

Directions:
1. Brown meat in a pan over medium heat.
2. Add oil and onion to the pan with meat. Mix well and cook over medium heat.
3. In a small bowl, mix together soy sauce, ginger, and garlic.
4. Add soy sauce mixture to the pan.
5. Add cabbage to the pan and toss to coat.
6. Add broth to the pan and mix well.
7. Cook over medium heat for 3 minutes.
8. Season with pepper and salt.
9. Garnish with green onion and serve.

Nutrition: Calories 171;Fat 5 g;Carbohydrates g;Sugar 5 g;Protein 23 g;Cholesterol 56 mg

Taco Chicken

Servings: 4
Cooking Time: 6 Hours
Ingredients:
* 1 lb chicken breasts, skinless and boneless
* 2 tbsp taco seasoning
* 1 cup chicken broth

Directions:
1. Place chicken in the slow cooker.
2. Mix together chicken broth and taco seasoning and pour over chicken.
3. Cover and cook on low for 6 hours.
4. Shred chicken using a fork.
5. Serve and enjoy.

Nutrition:Per Servings: Calories 233 Fat 8.7 g Carbohydrates 1.7 g Sugar 0.5 g Protein 34 g Cholesterol 101 mg

Baked Cod Cups

Servings: 12
Cooking Time: 30 Minutes
Ingredients:
* 1 pound cod fillets
* 1 tablespoon butter (melted)
* 1 garlic clove (minced)
* 1 cup almond flour
* 4 eggs (beaten)
* 1/4 cup plain unsweetened yogurt
* 1 teaspoon chopped fresh dill
* 1 lemon (zested, juiced)
* 1 teaspoon baking powder
* Salt and freshly ground black pepper, to taste

Directions:
1. Preheat oven to 375°F. Line wells of a muffin pan with foil liners and set aside.
2. Place cod fillets in a shallow microwave-safe dish. Brush about half of the butter over cod, sprinkle with garlic and cover dish. Micro-cook cod at high power for 3 minutes. Flip fillets, baste with butter and cook at high power until cod is flaky, 1 to minutes more.
3. Flake cod with a fork and mix with the juices from the microwave dish, almond flour, eggs, yogurt, dill, lemon juice and baking powder. Season cod mixture to taste with salt and pepper and stir until thoroughly combined.
4. Spoon cod mixture into prepared muffin pan and bake until cod cups are cooked through and lightly golden brown, about 25 minutes. Garnish cod cups with lemon juice and serve immediately. Enjoy!

Nutrition:Per Serving: Calories: 110; Total Fat: 4g; Saturated Fat: 1g; Protein: 16g; Carbs: 2g; Fiber: 0g; Sugar: 0g

Cucumber Tuna Salad

Servings: 6
Cooking Time: 5 Minutes
Ingredients:
* 2 cans tuna, drained

* 2/3 cup light mayonnaise
* 1 cup cucumber, diced
* 1/2 tsp dried dill
* 1 tsp fresh lemon juice
* Pepper
* Salt

Directions:
1. Add all ingredients into the mixing bowl and mix well.
2. Serve and enjoy.

Nutrition: Calories 215;Fat 15 g;Carbohydrates 6.9 g;Sugar 2 g;Protein 16.1 g;Cholesterol 25 mg

Avocado Eggs With Dried Rosemary

Servings: 6
Cooking Time: 20 Minutes
Ingredients:
* 3 medium ripe avocados, cut in half, and pit removed
* 6 large eggs
* 1 medium tomato, finely chopped
* 3 tbsp olive oil
* 2 tsp dried rosemary
* ¼ tsp salt
* ¼ tsp black pepper, ground

Directions:
1. Preheat oven to 350 degrees.
2. Cut avocado in half and remove the pit and flesh from the center. Place one boiled egg and chopped tomato in each avocado half and sprinkle with rosemary, salt and pepper.
3. Grease the baking pan with olive oil and place the avocados on top. You will want to use a small baking pan so your avocados can fit tightly. Place in the oven for about 15-20 minutes.
4. Remove from the oven and let it cool for a while before serving.

Nutrition:Per Serving: Net carbs 4 g;Fiber 2.4 g;Fats 16.g;Fatsr 4 g;Calories 185

One Sheet Pan Chicken Fried Rice

Servings: 4
Cooking Time: 15 Minutes
Ingredients:
- 2 - boneless skinless chicken breasts.
- Salt and pepper, to taste
- 1 15 - ounce can peas and carrots, drained
- ½ - white onion, diced
- 2 - eggs, whisked
- 2 - cups steamed white rice
- 3 - tablespoons sesame oil
- 1/3 - cup soy sauce
- Finely chopped green onions

Directions:
1. Oil an enormous preparing sheet and preheat stove to 375 degrees. Mastermind chicken pieces on the dish in a solitary layer so they aren't covering and season with salt and pepper to taste. Heat for 5 minutes.
2. Take the dish out from the stove, pour whisked eggs around the chicken pieces straightforwardly onto the container. Come back to broiler for 3-5 minutes until the egg is completely cooked. Utilize a fork or spatula to "scramble" the egg with the goal that it separates into little pieces.
3. Include rice and peas, carrots and white onions to the container and hurl all fixings so they are equitably appropriated. Shower sesame oil and soy sauce over everything and hurl once more. Sprinkle cleaved onions over the top.
4. Prepare for 5 minutes longer. Chicken ought to be cooked through and rice should start to darker on the base of the dish.
5. Toss all fixings once again and serve right away.
Nutrition: Calories: 24carbs: 24g;fat: 6g;protein: 28g

Stir-fried Chicken With Corn And Millet

Servings:1
Cooking Time: 15 Minutes
Ingredients:
- 3 - ounces boneless, skinless chicken thighs, cut into 1-inch pieces
- Salt
- Pepper
- ½ - tablespoon olive oil
- 2 - cloves garlic, sliced thin
- ½ - cup fresh corn kernels
- 2/3 - cup cooked millet
- 2 - tablespoons fresh parsley, chopped
- ¼ - lime, juiced
- ¼ - medium-size ripe avocado, chopped into ½ - inch pieces

Directions:
1. Season hen on all facets with salt and pepper. In a massive skillet over medium warmth, heat olive oil. Include chook and garlic and prepare dinner, blending sometimes, until fowl is cooked via, around 4minutes.
2. Include corn and prepare dinner, blending, just until it begins to mellow, round inutes greater.
3. Include millet, parsley, and juice. Cook, blending till warmed thru. Top with avocado.
Nutrition: Calories 537;fat 20g;carbs 66g;sugar 5g;protein 27g

Parmesan Spaghetti Squash

Servings: 4
Cooking Time: 45 To 50 Minutes
Ingredients:
- 1 large spaghetti squash
- 1 teaspoon olive oil
- Salt and freshly ground black pepper, to taste
- 1/2 cup marinara sauce
- 1 teaspoon garlic powder
- 1 teaspoon garlic salt
- 1/2 cup finely grated Parmesan cheese

Directions:
1. Preheat oven to 400°F.
2. Cut squash in half lengthwise and scoop out the seeds. Brush cut surfaces of squash with olive oil and season to taste with salt and pepper.
3. Place squash halves cut-sides down on a rimmed baking sheet and bake until tender, 45 to 50 minutes.
4. Scrape squash into strands from the peels with a fork. Toss squash strands with marinara sauce, garlic powder and onion powder and sprinkle with Parmesan cheese to serve. Enjoy!
Nutrition:Per Serving: Calories: 102; Total Fat: ; Saturated Fat: 2g; Protein: 5g Carbs: 8g; Fiber: 5g; Sugar: 2g

Southwestern Black Bean Cakes With Guacamole

Servings: 4
Cooking Time: 25 Minutes
Ingredients:
- 1 c. Whole wheat bread crumbs
- 3 tbsps. Chopped cilantro
- 2 garlic cloves
- 15 oz. Black beans
- 7 oz. Chipotle peppers in adobo sauce
- 1 tsp. Ground cumin
- 1 large egg
- ½ diced avocado
- 1 tbsp. Lime juice
- 1 tomato plum

Directions:
1. Drain beans and add all ingredients, except avocado, lime juice and eggs, to a food processor and run until the mixture begins to pull away from the sides.
2. Transfer to a large bowl and add egg, then mix well.
3. Form into 4 even patties and cook on a preheated, greased grill over medium heat for about 10 minutes, flipping halfway through.

4.   Add avocado and lime juice in a small bowl, then stir and mash together using a fork.
5.   Season to taste then serve with bean cakes.
Nutrition: Calories: 178, Fat: 7g, Carbs: 25g, Protein: 11g

Fresh Shrimp Spring Rolls

Servings: 12
Cooking Time: 20 Minutes
Ingredients:
- 12 sheets rice paper
- 12 bib lettuce
- 12 basil laves
- ¾ c. Cilantro
- 1 c. Shredded carrots
- ½ sliced cucumber
- 20 oz. Cooked shrimp

Directions:
1.   Add all vegetables and shrimp to separate bowls.
2.   Set a damp paper towel tower flat on work surface.
3.   Quickly wet a sheet of rice papers under warm water and lay on paper towel.
4.   Top with 1 of each vegetable and pieces of shrimp, then roll in rice paper into a burrito – like roll.
5.   Repeat until all vegetables and shrimp has been used up. Serve and enjoy.
Nutrition: Calories: , Fat: 2.9g, Carbs: 7.4g, Protein: 2.6g

Beef Recipes

Beef Stew With Rutabaga And Carrots

Servings:6
Cooking Time: 40 Minutes
Ingredients:
- 4 teaspoons extra-virgin olive oil, divided
- 1 pound beef sirloin steak, cut into 1-inch cubes
- 2 teaspoons minced garlic
- 1 medium onion, chopped
- 1 pound rutabaga, peeled, and cut into ½-inch cubes
- 3 medium carrots, peeled, and cut into ½-inch cubes
- 1 small tomato, diced
- 1 teaspoon smoked paprika
- ½ teaspoon ground coriander
- ¼ teaspoon red pepper flakes
- 2 tablespoons whole-wheat flour
- ½ cup red wine
- 3 cups low-sodium beef broth
- Fresh minced parsley, for garnish
- Post-Op
- 1 cup

Directions:
1. In a large soup pot or Dutch oven, heat 2 teaspoons of olive oil over medium heat.
2. Add the beef and brown it on all sides, stirring frequently, until no longer pink, about 5 minutes. Transfer to a bowl and set aside.
3. In the same pot, heat the remaining 2 teaspoons of olive oil over medium heat. Add the garlic and onion, and cook, stirring frequently, until the onion is tender, 1 to 2 minutes.
4. Stir in the rutabaga, carrots, tomato, paprika, coriander, and red pepper flakes.
5. Add the flour and cook, stirring constantly, for 1 minute. Add the red wine and stir for an additional minute.
6. Add the broth and return the beef to the pot. Bring to a boil and then reduce the heat to low to simmer. The sauce should start to thicken. Cover the pot and cook for 30 minutes, or until all the vegetables are tender.
7. Serve garnished with the parsley.
Nutrition: Per Serving (1 cup): Calories: 224; Total Fat: 10g; Protein: 17g; Carbs: 13g; Fiber: 3g; Sugars: 5g; Sodium: 139 mg

Spaghetti Squash Casserole With Ground Beef

Servings:8
Cooking Time: 75 Minutes
Ingredients:
- Nonstick cooking spray
- 2 medium spaghetti squash (2½ to 3 pounds)
- 1 pound supreme lean ground beef
- 1 large onion, minced
- 2 teaspoons minced garlic
- 1 (8-ounce) can tomato sauce
- 1 (10-ounce) can diced tomatoes
- 1 teaspoon dried basil
- 1 teaspoon dried oregano
- 1 cup shredded mozzarella cheese
- ½ cup shredded Parmigiano-Reggiano cheese
- Post-Op
- 1 cup serving

Directions:
1. Preheat the oven to 350°F. Coat a baking sheet with the cooking spray.
2. Halve the spaghetti squash, remove and discard the stem, pulp, and seeds, and place the halves cut-side down on the baking sheet. Bake for about 35 minutes, or until the flesh is tender.
3. While the squash bakes, spray a large skillet with the cooking spray, and place it over medium heat. Add the ground beef, onion, and garlic, and sauté for about 10 minutes, or until the beef is no longer pink and the onion is tender. Add the tomato sauce, diced tomatoes, basil, and oregano and stir to combine well. Remove the pan from the heat and set aside.
4. When the spaghetti squash is cool enough to handle, carefully use a fork to pull the flesh from the outer skin and make "spaghetti." Set aside in a bowl.
5. In a 9-by-13-inch baking dish, layer one-third of the meat-and-tomato mixture in the bottom of the dish. Evenly spread half of the squash over the meat layer. Layer another one-third of the meat mixture over the squash. Finish the last layer with the second half of the squash and the last one-third of the meat mixture. Sprinkle the mozzarella and Parmigiano-Reggiano cheeses over the top.
6. Cover with aluminum foil and bake for 30 minutes. Remove the foil and bake for 10 minutes more, or until the cheese begins to brown. Serve.
Nutrition: Per Serving (1 cup): Calories: 229; Total fat: 10g; Protein: 20g; Carbs: 16g; Fiber: 3g; Sugar: 11g; Sodium: 511mg

Italian Beef Sandwiches

Servings:6 Sandwiches
Cooking Time: 7 Hours
Ingredients:
- 1 cup water
- 1 tablespoon balsamic vinegar
- ¾ teaspoon garlic powder
- ¾ teaspoon onion powder
- 1½ teaspoons dried parsley
- ¾ teaspoon dried oregano
- ¼ teaspoon dried thyme
- ½ teaspoon dried basil
- ¼ teaspoon freshly ground black pepper
- 1½ pounds boneless beef chuck roast, fat trimmed
- 1 medium onion, sliced
- 1 red bell pepper, cut into strips
- 6 sprouted-grain hot dog buns or sandwich thins
- 1 (16-ounce) jar pepperoncini (optional)
- Post-Op
- 1 sandwich

Directions:
1. In a small bowl mix together the water, balsamic vinegar, garlic powder, onion powder, parsley, oregano, thyme, basil, and black pepper.
2. Place the beef in the slow cooker and add the onion and bell pepper.
3. Pour the sauce over the roast. Cover the slow cooker and cook on low for 7 hours. The meat should be tender and cooked through.
4. Carefully transfer the roast to a cutting board.
5. Thinly slice the roast.
6. Toast the buns or sandwich thins.
7. Layer each bun with the beef and top with the au jus, pepper, and onion. Serve with pepperoncini (if using).

Nutrition: Per Serving (1 sandwich): Calories: 351; Total fat: 9g; Protein: 31g; Carbs: 30g; Fiber: 5g; Sugar: 5g; Sodium: 41g

Mom's Sloppy Joes

Servings:8
Cooking Time: 30 Minutes
Ingredients:
- Nonstick cooking spray
- 1½ pounds supreme lean ground beef
- 1 cup chopped onion
- 1 cup chopped celery
- 1 (8-ounce) can tomato sauce
- ⅓ cup catsup (free of high-fructose corn syrup)
- 2 tablespoons white vinegar
- 2 tablespoons Worcestershire sauce
- 2 tablespoons Dijon mustard
- 1 tablespoon brown sugar
- Post-Op
- ¾ cup sloppy joe

Directions:
1. Spray a large skillet with the cooking spray, and place it over medium heat. Add the beef and brown until it is no longer pink, about 10 minutes. Drain off any grease.
2. Mix in the onion and celery, and cook for 2 to 3 minutes.
3. Stir in the tomato sauce, catsup, vinegar, Worcestershire sauce, mustard, and brown sugar. Bring the liquid to a simmer, and reduce the heat to low. Cook for 15 minutes, or until the sauce has thickened.
4. Spoon about ¾ cup of the sloppy joe mixture onto each plate, and serve.

Nutrition: Per Serving (¾ cup): Calories: 269; Total fat: ; Protein: 24g; Carbs: 32g; Fiber: 6g; Sugar: 6g; Sodium: 656mg

Creamy Beef Stroganoff With Mushrooms

Servings:6
Cooking Time: 30 Minutes
Ingredients:
- Nonstick cooking spray
- 1½ pounds extra-lean beef sirloin, cut into ½-inch strips
- 1 teaspoon extra-virgin olive oil
- 1 medium onion, chopped
- ½ pound mushrooms, sliced
- 2 tablespoon whole-wheat flour
- 1 cup low-sodium beef broth
- 1 cup water
- 1 teaspoon Worcestershire sauce
- ½ teaspoon dried thyme
- ½ teaspoon dried dill
- ½ cup low-fat plain Greek yogurt
- 2 tablespoons finely chopped fresh parsley, for garnish
- Post-Op
- 4 ounces

Directions:
1. Coat a medium pan with the cooking spray and place over medium-high heat. Add the beef. Cook, stirring frequently, until browned, about 5 minutes. Transfer to a bowl and set aside.
2. In the same pan, heat the olive oil over medium-high heat. Add the onion and cook until tender, 1 to 2 minutes.
3. Add the mushrooms and cook until tender, about 3 minutes.
4. Mix in the flour and stir to coat the onion and mushrooms.
5. Stir in the broth, water, Worcestershire sauce, thyme, dill. Bring to a boil, cover the pan, and cook for about 10 minutes, stirring frequently.
6. Stir in the yogurt. Mix in the beef. Serve, garnished with the parsley.

Nutrition: Per Serving (4 ounces): Calories: 351; Total fat: 9g; Protein: 31g; Carbs: 30g; Fiber: 5g; Sugar: 5g; Sodium: 418mg

Poultry Recipes

Egg Roll In A Bowl

Servings:6
Cooking Time: 20 Minutes
Ingredients:
- 2 teaspoons sesame oil, divided
- 1 teaspoon minced garlic
- 1 onion, finely diced
- 1 pound extra-lean ground chicken or turkey
- 1½ tablespoons low-sodium soy sauce or Bragg Liquid Aminos
- ½ cup low-sodium beef broth
- 2 teaspoons ground ginger
- ½ teaspoon freshly ground black pepper
- 4 cups green cabbage, chopped or shredded into 1-inch ribbons
- 1½ cups shredded carrots
- 1 cup fresh bean sprouts or 1 (14-ounce) can, drained and rinsed
- 2 scallions, finely chopped, for garnish
- Post-Op
- ¾ cup

Directions:
1. Place a large skillet over medium-high heat. Add 1 teaspoon of sesame oil and the garlic. Stir for 1 minute. Add the onion and cook until tender, 1 to 2 minutes. Add the ground chicken. Cook until browned, breaking up the meat into smaller pieces, 7 to 9 minutes.
2. While the meat is browning, mix together the remaining 1 teaspoon of the sesame oil, soy sauce, broth, ginger, and black pepper in a small bowl.
3. When the chicken is cooked, stir the sauce into the skillet. Add the cabbage, carrots, and bean sprouts. Stir to combine. Cover the skillet and simmer until the cabbage is tender, 5 to 7 minutes.
4. Serve in a bowl and garnish with the scallions and additional soy sauce to taste.

Nutrition: Per Serving (¾ cup): Calories: 133; Total fat: 3g; Protein: 19g; Carbs: 7g; Fiber 2g; Sugars: 4g; Sodium: 3mg

Chicken Caprese

Servings: 4
Cooking Time: 15 Minutes
Ingredients:
- 1 pound boneless skinless chicken breasts
- 2 tablespoons olive oil, divided
- 1 teaspoon garlic powder
- 1 teaspoon onion powder
- 1 teaspoon Italian herb seasoning
- Salt and freshly ground black pepper
- 1/2 cup grated mozzarella cheese
- 1 cup halved cherry tomatoes
- 2 tablespoons balsamic vinegar
- 2 tablespoons sliced fresh basil leaves

Directions:

1. Cut chicken breasts lengthwise into thick slices and brush all over with about 1 tablespoon olive oil. Mix garlic powder, onion powder and herb seasoning, sprinkle over chicken and season to taste with salt and pepper.
2. Heat remaining 1 tablespoon olive oil in a large nonstick skillet over medium heat and cook chicken until lightly golden brown and no longer pink inside, 8 to 10 minutes, turning as necessary. Sprinkle mozzarella cheese over chicken and cook until cheese is melted, about 1 minute more.
3. Transfer chicken to a serving plate and arrange tomatoes over chicken. Drizzle balsamic vinegar over chicken, sprinkle with basil and serve immediately. Enjoy!

Nutrition:Per Serving: Net carbs 3 g;Fiber 1 g;Fats 9 g;Fatsr g;Calories 170

Chicken Thighs

Servings: 6
Cooking Time: 40 Minutes
Ingredients:
- 2 lbs. chicken thighs
- 2 medium onions, chopped
- 2 small chili peppers
- 1 cup chicken broth
- ¼ cup freshly squeezed orange juice, unsweetened
- 1 tsp orange extract, sugar-free
- 2 tbsp olive oil
- 1 tsp barbecue seasoning mix
- 1 small red onion, chopped

Directions:
1. Heat up the olive oil in a large saucepan. Add chopped onions and fry for several minutes, over a medium temperature – until golden color.
2. Combine chili peppers, orange juice and orange extract. Mix well in a food processor for -30 seconds. Add this mixture into a saucepan and stir well. Reduce heat to simmer.
3. Coat the chicken with barbecue seasoning mix and put into a saucepan. Add chicken broth and bring it to boil. Cook over a medium temperature until the water evaporates. Remove from the heat.
4. Preheat the oven to 350 degrees. Place the chicken into a large baking dish. Bake for about 15 minutes to get a nice crispy, golden brown color.

Nutrition:Per Serving: Net carbs 2 g;Fiber 0.9 g;Fats 16.2 g;Fatsr 3 g;Calories 357

Slow Cooker White Chicken Chili

Servings:6
Cooking Time: 6 Hours
Ingredients:
- 2 (14.5-ounce) cans chickpeas, drained and rinsed, divided
- 2 cups low-sodium chicken broth, divided
- 1 pound boneless, skinless chicken breasts
- 1 large onion, diced
- 1 jalapeño pepper, seeded, minced
- 1 tablespoon ground cumin
- 1½ teaspoons ground coriander
- 2 teaspoons dried oregano
- 2 teaspoons chili powder
- 1 (4-ounce) can diced green chiles
- 2 cups water
- ¼ cup chopped cilantro, for garnish (optional)
- Post-Op
- ¼ cup (2 ounces)
- ½ cup (4 ounces)
- 4 ounces

Directions:
1. Prepare bean puree. In a blender or food processor, blend 1 can of the beans with 1 cup of broth. Set aside.
2. Place the chicken breasts in a 4- or 6-quart slow cooker. Top them with the onion, jalapeño, cumin, coriander, oregano, chili powder, and green chiles.
3. Add the remaining 1 cup of broth, water, remaining 1 can of beans, and bean puree.
4. Cover the slow cooker, turn on low, and set the timer for 6 hours. At the 5½-hour mark, transfer the chicken to a plate and shred it with a fork. Return it to the slow cooker, and continue cooking on low for an additional 20 to 30 minutes before serving, allowing the chicken to absorb some of the liquid.
5. Ladle into bowls to serve and garnish with the cilantro.
Nutrition: Per Serving (1 cup): Calories: 225; Total fat: 3g; Protein: 2; Carbs: 25g; Fiber: 7g; Sugar: 3g; Sodium: 661mg

Grilled Chicken Wings

Servings: 6
Cooking Time: 20 Minutes
Ingredients:
- 1 and ½ pounds frozen chicken wings
- Fresh ground black pepper
- 1 teaspoon garlic powder
- 1 cup buffalo

Directions:
1. Pre-heat your grill to 350 degrees F.
2. Season wings with pepper and garlic powder, grill wings for 15 minutes per side.
3. Once they are browned and crispy, toss grilled wings in Buffalo wings sauce and olive oil.
4. Enjoy!

Nutrition: Per Serving:;Net carbs 1 g;Fiber 3 g;Fats 6 g;Fatsr 2 g;Calories 82

Lemon Chicken

Servings: 3
Cooking Time: 20 Minutes
Ingredients:
- 2 teaspoons olive oil
- 2 boneless skinless chicken breasts
- 2 garlic cloves, minced
- 1 cup chicken stock
- 2 lemons, zested, juiced
- 1 teaspoon lemon pepper seasoning
- 1/2 teaspoon dried basil
- 1/2 teaspoon dried oregano
- Salt and freshly ground black pepper
- 1 tablespoon cornstarch
- 2 tablespoons cold water

Directions:
1. Heat olive oil in a large nonstick skillet over medium heat and sauté chicken just until cooked through, 7 to 8 minutes, stirring frequently.
2. Add garlic and sauté about 1 minute more, stirring constantly.Add chicken stock, lemon juice, lemon pepper, basil and oregano to chicken mixture and season to taste with salt and pepper. Reduce heat and simmer until chicken is cooked through and liquid is slightly reduced, 7 to 8 minutes, stirring occasionally.
3. Whisk cornstarch into cold water, add to skillet and stir gently until combined. Simmer until sauce is thickened, about 2 minutes, stirring constantly.
4. Transfer lemon chicken to a large bowl, sprinkle with lemon zest and serve immediately. Enjoy!
Nutrition:Per Serving: Net carbs 8 g;Fiber 1 g;Fats g;Fatsr 2 g;Calories 134

Creamy Chicken Soup With Cauliflower

Servings:8 Cup
Cooking Time: 40 Minutes
Ingredients:
- 1 teaspoon minced garlic
- 1 teaspoon extra-virgin olive oil
- ½ yellow onion, diced
- 1 carrot, diced
- 1 celery stalk, diced
- 1½ pounds (3 or 4 medium) cooked chicken breast, diced
- 2 cups low-sodium chicken broth
- 2 cups water
- 1 teaspoon freshly ground black pepper
- 1 teaspoon dried thyme
- 2½ cups fresh cauliflower florets
- 1 cup fresh spinach, chopped
- 2 cups nonfat or 1% milk
- Post-Op
- 1 cup serving

Directions:
1. Place a large soup pot over medium-high heat. Sauté the garlic in the olive oil for 1 minute.
2. Add the onion, carrot, and celery and sauté until tender, 3 to 5 minutes.
3. Add the chicken breast, broth, water, black pepper, thyme, and cauliflower. Bring to a simmer, reduce the heat to medium-low, and cook, uncovered, for 30 minutes.
4. Add the fresh spinach and stir until wilted, about 5 minutes.
5. Stir in the milk, then serve immediately.

Nutrition: Per Serving (1 cup): Calories: 1; Total fat: 3g; Protein: 25g; Carbs: 5g; Fiber: 1g; Sugar: 4g; Sodium: 54mg

Mediterranean Turkey Meatloaf

Servings:4
Cooking Time: 55 Minutes
Ingredients:
- For the meatloaf
- Nonstick cooking spray
- 1 pound extra-lean ground turkey
- 1 large egg, lightly beaten
- ¼ cup whole-wheat bread crumbs
- ¼ fat-free feta cheese
- ¼ cup Kalamata olives, pitted and halved
- ¼ cup chopped fresh parsley
- ¼ cup minced red onion
- ¼ cup plus 2 tablespoons hummus, such as Lantana Cucumber Hummus, divided
- 2 teaspoons minced garlic
- ½ teaspoon dried basil
- ¼ teaspoon dried oregano
- For the topping
- ½ small cucumber, peeled, seeded, and chopped
- 1 large tomato, chopped
- 2 to 3 tablespoons minced fresh basil
- Juice of ½ lemon
- 1 teaspoon extra-virgin olive oil
- Post-Op
- 2 ounces
- 2 to 4 ounces

Directions:
1. TO MAKE THE MEATLOAF
2. 1 Preheat the oven to 350°F. Coat an 8-by-4-inch loaf pan with the cooking spray.
3. 2 In a large bowl, combine the ground turkey, egg, bread crumbs, feta cheese, olives, parsley, onion, 2 tablespoons of hummus, garlic, basil, and oregano. Using clean hands, mix until just combined.
4. 3 Place the meatloaf mixture evenly in the loaf pan. Spread the remaining ¼ cup of hummus over the top of the meatloaf.
5. 4 Bake for minutes.
6. TO MAKE THE TOPPING
7. 1 In a small bowl, mix together the cucumber, tomato, basil, lemon juice, and olive oil. Refrigerate until ready to serve.
8. 2 The meatloaf is done when it reaches an internal temperature of 165°F. Let it sit for 5 minutes before serving, then slice and garnish with the topping

Nutrition: Per Serving (4 ounces): Calories: 232; Total fat: 8g; Protein: 31g; Carbs: 10g; Fiber: 2g; Sugar: 2g; Sodium: 370mg

Chicken Cauliflower Bowls

Servings: 4
Cooking Time: 12 Minutes
Ingredients:
- 1 large head cauliflower, cored
- 1/2 cup chicken stock
- 1 teaspoon butter
- 1/4 cup chopped onion
- 1/4 cup chopped bell pepper
- 1 cup chopped cooked chicken breast
- 1 teaspoon garlic powder
- Salt and freshly ground black pepper, to taste
- 1/4 cup shredded white cheddar cheese

Directions:
1. Pour water into a large saucepan to a depth of about 2 inches. Set steamer basket in saucepan and place cauliflower in basket. Cover pan and steam over medium heat until cauliflower is soft, to 12 minutes.
2. Meanwhile, heat butter in a medium nonstick skillet and sauté onion and bell pepper until softened, 4 to 5 minutes, stirring frequently. Remove skillet from heat, add cooked chicken and garlic powder, season to taste with salt and pepper and stir to combine.
3. Carefully remove cauliflower from steamer basket and place in a large bowl. Crumble and lightly mash cauliflower with a fork and season to taste with salt and pepper. Add chicken stock to cauliflower and puree with an immersion blender until smooth, adding more stock if needed.
4. Scoop cauliflower into bowls, top with the chicken mixture and sprinkle with the grated cheese to serve. Enjoy!

Nutrition:Per Serving: Net carbs 13 g;Fiber 6 g;Fats g;Fatsr 4 g;Calories 149

Zoodles With Turkey Meatballs

Servings:4
Cooking Time: 20 Minutes
Ingredients:
- Nonstick cooking spray
- 1 large egg
- ½ cup whole-wheat bread crumbs
- ⅓ cup chopped onion
- ½ teaspoon freshly ground black pepper
- 1 pound extra-lean ground turkey
- 1 pound zucchini (about 3 medium zucchini)
- 1 teaspoon extra-virgin olive oil
- 2 cups Marinara Sauce with Italian Herbs, or a low-sugar jarred marinara sauce
- Post-Op
- 1 meatball with 2 ounces sauce
- 2 meatballs with 2 to 4 ounces sauce and ¼ cup zoodles

Directions:
1. Preheat the oven to 400°F. Coat the bottom of a shallow baking pan with the cooking spray.
2. In a large bowl, combine the egg, bread crumbs, onion, and pepper.
3. Add the ground turkey and using clean hands, mix well until the mixture is evenly distributed.
4. Shape the meat mixture into 2-inch balls and place in the baking pan.
5. Bake, uncovered, for 15 minutes.
6. Cut off the ends of the zucchini. Use a mandolin, spiralizer, or the side of a box grater to slice the zucchini into long, thin strips.
7. In a medium skillet over medium heat, heat the olive oil. Add the zucchini strips and sauté for about 5 minutes, or until tender. Transfer to a serving bowl.
8. Serve the meatballs over the zoodles and top with the marinara sauce.

Nutrition: Per Serving (2 meatballs with 2 ounces sauce and ¼ cup zoodles): Calories: 1; Total fat: 5g; Protein: 22g; Carbs: 15g; Fiber: 3g; Sugar: 4g; Sodium: 205mg

Chicken Cordon Bleu

Servings: 5
Cooking Time: 30 Minutes
Ingredients:
- 6 chicken breasts, skinless, boneless, thinly sliced
- 6 slices lean deli ham
- 6 slices reduced-fat Swiss cheese, halved
- 2 large eggs
- 1 tablespoon water½ cup whole wheat bread crumbs
- 2 tablespoons Parmigiano-Reggiano cheese

Directions:
1. Pre-heat your oven to 450 degrees F.
2. Spray a baking sheet with cooking spray, pound chicken breasts to ¼ inch thickness.
3. Layer 1 slice ham and 1 slice (2 halves) cheese on each chicken breast.
4. Roll chicken and transfer them to the baking sheet (seam side down).
5. Take a small bowl and add whisk in eggs, take another bowl and mix in bread crumbs and cheese.
6. Use a pastry brush and lightly brush each chicken roll with egg wash. Sprinkle bread crumbs all over.
7. Bake for 30 minutes until the top is lightly browned.
8. Enjoy!

Nutrition:Per Serving: Net carbs 3 g;Fiber 1 g;Fats 7 g;Fatsr 4 g;Calories 174

Slow Cooker Turkey Chili

Servings:16
Cooking Time: 8 Hours
Ingredients:
- Nonstick cooking spray
- 2 pounds extra-lean ground turkey
- 2 (14.5-ounce) cans kidney beans, drained and rinsed
- 1 (28-ounce) can diced tomatoes with green chiles
- 1 (8-ounce) can tomato puree
- 1 large onion, finely chopped
- 1 green bell pepper, finely chopped
- 2 celery stalks, finely chopped
- 4 teaspoons minced garlic
- 1 teaspoon dried oregano
- 2 tablespoons ground cumin
- 3 tablespoons chili powder
- 1 (8-ounce) can tomato juice
- Post-Op
- ¼ cup
- ¼ to ½ cup
- ½ to 1 cup

Directions:
1. Place a large skillet over medium-high heat and coat it with the cooking spray. Add the ground turkey. Using a wooden spoon, break it into smaller pieces and cook until browned, 7 to 9 minutes.
2. While the turkey browns, place the beans, tomatoes, tomato puree, onion, bell pepper, celery, garlic, oregano, cumin, chili powder, and tomato juice in the slow cooker. Stir in the cooked ground turkey and mix well.
3. Cover the slow cooker and turn on low to cook for 8 hours.
4. Serve garnished with Greek yogurt, shredded Cheddar cheese, and chopped scallions (if using).

Nutrition: Per Serving (½ cup): Calories: 140; Total fat: 4g; Protein: 14g; Carbs: 12g; Fiber: 4g; Sugar: 4g; Sodium: 280mg

Whole Herbed Roasted Chicken In The Slow Cooker

Servings:6
Cooking Time: 7 Hours
Ingredients:
- 1 teaspoon garlic powder
- 1 teaspoon smoked paprika
- 1 teaspoon onion powder
- 1 teaspoon dried thyme
- ½ teaspoon freshly ground black pepper
- ½ teaspoon dried sage
- 1 (4-pound) whole chicken
- 2 sprigs fresh rosemary
- 2 lemon wedges
- Post-Op
- ¼ cup (2 ounces)
- ½ cup (4 ounces)
- ½ to ¾ cup (4 to 6 ounces)

Directions:
1. In a small bowl, mix together the garlic powder, paprika, onion powder, thyme, black pepper, and sage.
2. Remove any giblets from the chicken cavity. Rinse the outside and inner cavity of the chicken under cold water and use a paper towel to pat dry. Place the chicken in the slow cooker.
3. Rub the chicken with the herb mixture, getting as much as possible under the skin.
4. Stuff the inside of the chicken with the rosemary and lemon wedges.
5. Cover the slow cooker and turn on low to cook for 7 hours, or until the temperature of the innermost part of a thigh and thickest part of the breast has reached 165°F.

Nutrition: Per Serving (4 ounces): Calories: 191; Total fat: 8g; Protein: 29g; Carbs: 0g; Fiber: 0g; Sugar: 0g; Sodium: 8g

Dz's Grilled Chicken Wings

Servings:about 18 Wings
Cooking Time: 20 Minutes
Ingredients:
- 1½ pounds frozen chicken wings
- Freshly ground black pepper
- 1 teaspoon garlic powder
- 1 cup buffalo wing sauce, such as Frank's RedHot
- 1 teaspoon extra-virgin olive oil
- Post-Op
- 2 or 3 wings

Directions:
1. Preheat the grill to 350°F.
2. Season the wings with the black pepper and garlic powder.
3. Grill the wings for 15 minutes per side. They will be browned and crispy when finished.
4. Toss the grilled wings in the buffalo wing sauce and olive oil.
5. Serve immediately.

Nutrition: Per Serving (1 wing): Calories: 82; Total fat: ; Protein: 7g; Carbs: 1g; Fiber: 0g; Sugar: 0g; Sodium: 400mg

Turkey Soup

Servings: 6
Cooking Time: 30 Minutes
Ingredients:
- 1 tablespoon butter
- 1 pound boneless skinless turkey thighs
- 6 cups chicken stock
- 1/2 teaspoon kosher salt, plus more to taste
- 1/4 teaspoon freshly ground black pepper
- 2 celery stalks, diced
- 2 carrots, peeled, diced
- 1 small onion, diced
- 1 1/2 teaspoons dried Italian herb seasoning
- 2 dried bay leaves

Directions:
1. Melt butter in a stock pot or large saucepan over medium heat and sauté turkey thighs until browned on all sides, about 5 minutes.
2. Add chicken stock, salt and pepper to pot and heat to a boil. Reduce heat, cover pot and simmer for about 10 minutes.
3. Add celery, carrots, onion, herb seasoning and bay leaves to pot, season to taste with salt and pepper and stir to combine. Cover pot and simmer until vegetables are tender, about 15 minutes more.
4. Remove bay leaves from soup and discard. Remove turkey thighs from soup, cut into bite-size pieces and stir back into soup. Serve soup immediately and enjoy!

Nutrition:Per Serving: Net carbs 4 g;Fiber 1 g;Fats 7 g;Fatsr 4 g;Calories 139

Mexican Taco Skillet With Red Peppers And Zucchini

Servings:6
Cooking Time: 20 Minutes
Ingredients:
- 2 teaspoons extra-virgin olive oil
- 1 large onion, finely chopped
- 1 tablespoon minced garlic
- 1 jalapeño pepper, seeded and finely chopped
- 2 medium red bell peppers, diced
- 1 pound boneless, skinless chicken breast, cut into 1-inch cubes
- 1 tablespoon ground cumin
- 1 teaspoon low-sodium taco seasoning, such as from Penzeys Spices
- 1 (14.5-ounce) can diced tomatoes
- 1 large zucchini, halved lengthwise and diced
- ½ cup shredded mild Cheddar cheese
- 1 cup chopped fresh cilantro
- ½ cup chopped scallions
- Post-Op
- 1 cup

Directions:
1. In a large skillet over medium heat, heat the olive oil. Add the onion, garlic, jalapeño, and red bell peppers. Sauté the vegetables for about 5 minutes, or until tender.
2. Add the chicken, cumin, and taco seasoning, and stir until the chicken and vegetables are well coated.
3. Stir in the tomatoes. Bring the mixture to a boil. Cover the skillet, reduce the heat to medium-low, and cook for 10 minutes.
4. Add the zucchini and mix well. Cook for 7 minutes more, or until the zucchini is tender.
5. Remove the skillet from the heat. Mix in the cheese, cilantro, and scallions, and serve.
Nutrition: Per Serving (1 cup): Calories: 1; Total fat: 7g; Protein: 18g; Carbs: 8g; Fiber: 2g; Sugar: 5g; Sodium: 261mg

Baked Potato Soup

Servings:6
Cooking Time: 30 Minutes
Ingredients:
- 4 slices turkey bacon (nitrate-free)
- 2 tablespoons extra-virgin olive oil
- 3 tablespoons whole-wheat flour
- 1½ cups 1% milk
- 1½ cups vegetable or chicken broth
- 3 medium unpeeled russet potatoes, cut into 1-inch chunks
- ½ cup low-fat plain Greek yogurt
- ½ cup shredded sharp Cheddar cheese
- 4 tablespoons chopped chives
- Post-Op
- ¼ cup
- ½ cup
- 1 to 2 cups

Directions:
1. Place a large stock pot over medium heat. Add the bacon and cook until crispy on both sides, turning once, about 5 minutes total. Transfer to a paper towel-lined plate to absorb any excess grease. Once cooled, chop finely and set aside.

2. Heat the olive oil in the stock pot over medium heat. Add the flour and cook, stirring constantly, until browned, 2 to 3 minutes. Add the milk and whisk constantly until it starts to thicken. Whisk in the broth.
3. Add the potatoes. Bring to a boil, then reduce the heat to low and let the soup simmer for about 20 minutes, or until the potatoes are tender.
4. Add the Greek yogurt and stir to combine.
5. Serve garnished with the turkey bacon, cheese, chives, and additional dollop of plain Greek yogurt.
Nutrition: Per Serving (1 cup): Calories: 181; Total fat: 9g; Protein: 9g; Carbs: 18g; Fiber: 3g; Sugar: 1g; Sodium: 174mg

Ranch-seasoned Crispy Chicken Tenders

Servings:6 Chicken Tenders
Cooking Time: 20 Minutes
Ingredients:
- Nonstick cooking spray
- 6 chicken tenderloin pieces (about 1¼ pounds)
- 2 tablespoons whole-wheat pastry flour
- 1 egg, lightly beaten
- ½ cup whole-wheat bread crumbs
- 2 tablespoons grated Parmigiano-Reggiano cheese
- 2 teaspoons dried parsley
- ¾ teaspoon dried dill
- ¼ teaspoon garlic powder
- ¼ teaspoon onion powder
- ¼ teaspoon dried basil
- ⅛ teaspoon freshly ground black pepper
- Post-Op
- 1 chicken tender

Directions:
1. Preheat the oven to 425°F. Spray a baking sheet with the cooking spray.
2. Prepare three small dishes for coating the chicken. Place the flour in one, the egg in the second, and in the last dish mix together the bread crumbs, Parmigiano-Reggiano cheese, parsley, dill, garlic powder, onion powder, basil, and black pepper.
3. Working one at a time, dip each tenderloin into the flour. Shake off any excess, then dip the chicken into the egg. Finally, place the tenderloin in the bread crumbs and press to coat in the mixture. Place on the baking sheet.
4. Bake for about 20 minutes, or until crispy, brown and cooked through. Serve immediately.
Nutrition: Per Serving (1 chicken tender): Calories: 162; Total fat: 2g; Protein: 2; Carbs: 8g; Fiber: 1g; Sugar: 1g; Sodium: 239mg

Baked "fried Chicken" Thighs

Servings:4
Cooking Time: 35 Minutes
Ingredients:
- Nonstick cooking spray
- 1 teaspoon smoked paprika
- ½ teaspoon garlic powder
- ½ teaspoon freshly ground black pepper
- ½ teaspoon cayenne pepper
- ½ teaspoon dried oregano
- 4 (5-ounce) boneless, skinless chicken thighs
- 2 large eggs
- 1 tablespoon water
- 1 teaspoon Dijon mustard
- 2½ cups bran flakes
- Post-Op
- ½ chicken thigh (2 to 4 ounces)
- 1 chicken thigh (4 to 6 ounces)

Directions:
1. Preheat the oven to 400°F. Line a large rimmed baking sheet with aluminum foil, and place it in the oven below a clean oven rack. Spray the clean rack with the cooking spray.
2. In a large zip-top bag, combine the paprika, garlic powder, black pepper, cayenne pepper, and oregano. Add the chicken thighs to the bag, seal the bag, and shake to coat the thighs with the seasonings. Set aside.
3. In a small bowl, lightly whisk together the eggs, water, and mustard.
4. Crush the bran flakes in another large plastic bag.
5. To bread the chicken, dredge the seasoned chicken thighs in the egg mixture, and then put them in the bag of crushed cereal. Shake to coat well.
6. Place the chicken thighs on the clean oven rack, making sure the baking sheet is directly under the chicken to catch any drippings.
7. Bake for 35 minutes, or until the thighs are crispy and reach an internal temperature of 165°F, and serve.
Nutrition: Per Serving (1 chicken thigh): Calories: 272; Total fat: ; Protein: 35g; Carbs: 15g; Fiber: 3g; Sugar: 3g; Sodium: 279mg

Creamy Chicken Soup And Cauliflower

Servings: 4
Cooking Time: 40 Minutes
Ingredients:
- 1 teaspoon garlic, minced
- 1 teaspoon extra virgin olive oil
- ½ yellow onion, diced1 carrot, diced
- 1 celery stalk, diced
- 1 and ½ pounds cooked chicken breast, diced
- 2 cups low sodium chicken broth
- 2 cups of water
- 1 teaspoon fresh ground black pepper
- 1 teaspoon dried thyme
- 2 and ½ cups fresh cauliflower florets
- 1 cup fresh spinach, chopped
- 2 cups nonfat milk

Directions:
1. Place large soup over medium-high heat and add garlic in olive oil, Sauté for minute.
2. Add onion, carrot, celery, Sauté for 3-5 minutes.
3. Add chicken breast, broth, water, pepper, thyme, cauliflower and simmer over low-medium heat, cover and cook for minutes.
4. Add fresh spinach and stir for 5 minutes.
5. Stir in milk and serve, enjoy!
Nutrition:Per Serving: Net carbs 5 g;Fiber 1 g;Fats 3 g;Fatsr 2 g;Calories 1

Cauliflower Pizza With Caramelized Onions And Chicken Sausage

Servings:1 (12-inch) Pizza
Cooking Time: 35 Minutes
Ingredients:
- 1 large head cauliflower, stemmed, with leaves removed
- 2 large eggs, lightly beaten
- 2 cups shredded part-skim mozzarella cheese, divided
- ½ cup shredded Parmigiano-Reggiano cheese
- ½ teaspoon dried oregano
- ¼ teaspoon dried basil
- ½ teaspoon garlic powder
- 2 teaspoons extra-virgin olive oil
- 2 red onions, thinly sliced
- 2 links precooked chicken sausage (nitrate-free), cut into ¼-inch rounds
- Post-Op
- 1 or 2 slices

Directions:
1. Preheat the oven to 400°F.
2. Cut the cauliflower head into 3 or 4 large pieces. Place in a food processor and pulse for 1 to 2 seconds at a time until all the pieces are the size of rice. Remove any large pieces that won't break down. Transfer the riced cauliflower to a bowl and pat dry with a paper towel.
3. Place a small pot over medium heat and add ½ cup water. Put the riced cauliflower directly in the pot (or in a steamer basket in the pot), and bring the water to a boil. Cover the pot and steam the cauliflower for 3 to 5 minutes, or until tender. Remove the pan from the heat and let cool. Place the steamed cauliflower on a paper towel to soak up any moisture and pat dry.
4. In a medium bowl, combine the eggs, 1 cup of mozzarella, Parmigiano-Reggiano cheese, oregano, basil, and garlic powder. Add the cauliflower and mix well.
5. Spread the cauliflower mixture onto a 12-inch round pizza pan, and press it into an even layer like a pizza crust. Press until it is less than 1-inch thick. Bake for 20 minutes.
6. While the crust bakes, place a large skillet over medium heat. Heat the olive oil and add the onions and cook, stirring occasionally, until caramelized, about 20 minutes.
7. Spread the caramelized onions and chicken sausage evenly across the cauliflower crust. Top with the remaining 1 cup of mozzarella cheese. Bake the pizza for 10 minutes more, or until the cheese is bubbly.
Nutrition: Per Serving (1 slice): Calories: 121; Total fat: 7g; Protein: 10g; Carbs: ; Fiber: 4g; Sugar: 3g; Sodium: 260mg

Chicken, Barley, And Vegetable Soup

Servings:8 Cups
Cooking Time: 50 Minutes
Ingredients:
- 1 tablespoon extra-virgin olive oil
- 1 teaspoon minced garlic
- 1 large onion, diced
- 2 large carrots, chopped
- 3 celery stalks, chopped
- 1 (14.5-ounce) can diced tomatoes
- ¾ cup pearl barley
- 2½ cups diced cooked chicken, such as leftovers from Whole Herbed Roasted Chicken in the Slow Cooker
- 4 cups low-sodium chicken broth
- 2 cups water
- ½ teaspoon dried thyme
- ½ teaspoon dried sage
- ¼ teaspoon dried rosemary
- 2 bay leaves
- Post-Op
- 1 cup

Directions:
1. Place a large soup pot over medium-high heat. Sauté the olive oil and garlic for 1 minute.
2. Add the onion, carrots, and celery and sauté until tender, 3 to 5 minutes.
3. Add the tomatoes, barley, chicken, broth, water, thyme, sage, rosemary, and bay leaves. Bring to a simmer, then reduce the heat to medium-low and cook, uncovered, for about 45 minutes. The soup is done when the barley is tender.
4. Remove and discard bay leaves before serving.
Nutrition: Per Serving (1 cup): Calories: 198; Total fat: 3g; Protein: 16g; Carbs: 9g; Fiber: 2g; Sugar: 3g; Sodium: 8mg

Chicken "nachos" With Sweet Bell Peppers

Servings:about 16 "nachos"
Cooking Time: 25 Minutes
Ingredients:
- Nonstick cooking spray
- 1 (1-pound) package mini bell peppers, stemmed, seeded, and halved
- 2 teaspoons extra-virgin olive oil
- ½ onion, minced
- 2 cups cooked shredded chicken breast (see Ingredient tip)
- 1 large tomato, diced
- 1 teaspoon garlic powder
- 1 teaspoon ground cumin
- ½ teaspoon smoked paprika
- 1 cup shredded Colby Jack cheese
- ¼ cup sliced black olives
- 3 scallions, finely sliced
- 1 jalapeño pepper, seeded, thinly sliced (optional)
- Post-Op
- 2 mini bell pepper halves

Directions:
1. Preheat the oven to 400°F. Line a baking sheet with aluminum foil and coat the foil with the cooking spray.
2. Arrange the bell pepper halves on the baking sheet cut-side up.
3. Heat the olive oil in a large skillet over medium heat. Add the onion and sauté for 1 to 2 minutes, or until tender. Add the chicken, tomato, garlic powder, cumin, and paprika and cook for about 5 minutes, or until the tomato has softened and the chicken is heated through.
4. Spoon 1 heaping tablespoon of the chicken mixture into each mini bell pepper half. Top each with the cheese, black olives, scallions, and jalapeño (if using).
5. Bake for 15 minutes, or until cheese has melted and browned. Enjoy immediately.
Nutrition: Per Serving (2 mini stuffed bell pepper halves): Calories: 189; Total fat: 3g; Protein: 29g; Carbs: 9g; Fiber: 2g; Sugar: 2g; Sodium: 143mg

Jerk Chicken With Mango Salsa

Servings:4
Cooking Time: 15 Minutes
Ingredients:
- 2 tablespoons extra-virgin olive oil
- Juice of 1 lime
- 1 tablespoon minced garlic
- 1 teaspoon ground ginger
- ½ teaspoon dried thyme
- ½ teaspoon cinnamon
- ½ teaspoon ground allspice
- ½ teaspoon ground nutmeg
- ¼ teaspoon cayenne pepper
- ¼ teaspoon ground cloves
- 1 teaspoon freshly ground black pepper
- 4 boneless, skinless chicken breasts about (1 pound chicken)
- 1 cup Mango Salsa
- Post-Op
- 4 ounces with ¼ cup Mango Salsa

Directions:
1. In a gallon-size zip-top freezer bag, put the olive oil, lime juice, garlic, ginger, thyme, cinnamon, allspice, nutmeg, cayenne, cloves, and black pepper. Tightly seal the bag and gently mix the marinade.
2. Add the chicken breasts to the marinade. Tightly seal the bag and shake to coat the chicken in the marinade.
3. Refrigerate for at least 30 minutes or overnight.
4. Preheat the grill to medium-high heat. Place the chicken on the grill and discard the marinade. Cook the chicken for about 6 minutes on each side or until the breasts are no longer pink in the middle and reach an internal temperature of 165°F. Alternatively, bake the chicken in a preheated 400°F oven for about 25 minutes, or until the juices run clear.
5. Let the chicken rest for 5 minutes before slicing. Top the chicken slices with the Mango Salsa.
Nutrition: Per Serving (4 ounces): Calories: 20 Total fat: 9g; Protein: 25g; Carbs: 11g; Fiber: 1g; Sugar: 9g; Sodium: 111mg

Chicken Curry Wraps

Servings: 2
Cooking Time: 10 Minutes
Ingredients:
- 1 cup cooked diced chicken
- 1/2 cup plain unsweetened yogurt
- 1 tablespoon skim milk, plus more if needed
- 1 celery stalk, diced
- 1/2 teaspoon curry powder
- 1/4 teaspoon onion powder
- Salt and freshly ground black pepper
- 2 large green lettuce leaves
- 1 tablespoon slivered almonds, toasted

Directions:
1. Mix chicken, yogurt, milk, celery, curry powder and onion powder and season to taste with salt and pepper.
2. Spread chicken mixture on lettuce leaves and sprinkle with almonds.
3. Roll up lettuce leaves burrito-style over chicken mixture. Serve immediately and enjoy!
Nutrition:Per Serving: Net carbs 3 g;Fiber 1 g;Fats 5 g;Fatsr 3 g;Calories 1

Buffalo Chicken Wrap

Servings: 4
Cooking Time: 10 Minutes
Ingredients:
- 3 cups rotisserie chicken breast
- 2 cups romaine lettuce, chopped
- 1 tomato, diced½ red onion, finely sliced
- ¼ cup buffalo wing sauce
- ¼ cup creamy peppercorn ranch dressing
- Chopped raw celery as for garnish
- 5 small whole grain low carb wraps

Directions:
1. Take a large mixing bowl and add chicken, lettuce, tomato, onion, wing sauce, dressing, and celery.

2. Add 1 cup of mixture onto each wrap and foil wrap over the salad.
3. Use a toothpick to secure the wrap, enjoy!
Nutrition:Per Serving: Net carbs 1g;Fiber 3 g;Fats 7 g;Fatsr 1 g;Calories 200

Slow Cooker Barbecue Shredded Chicken

Servings:4
Cooking Time: 6½ To 8½ Hours
Ingredients:
- 4 (4-ounce) boneless, skinless chicken breasts
- 1 cup catsup (free of high-fructose corn syrup)
- ½ cup water
- 1 tablespoon freshly squeezed lemon juice
- 1 tablespoon dried onions
- ½ teaspoon dried mustard
- ¼ teaspoon red pepper flakes
- 3 tablespoons Worcestershire sauce
- 1 tablespoon white vinegar
- Post-Op
- ¼ cup (2 ounces)
- ½ cup (4 ounces)
- ½ cup (4 ounces)

Directions:
1. Place the chicken breasts in a slow cooker.
2. In a small bowl, whisk together the catsup, water, lemon juice, dried onions, dried mustard, red pepper flakes, Worcestershire sauce, and white vinegar. Pour the mixture over the chicken.
3. Cover the slow cooker and turn on low to cook for 6 to 8 hours.
4. Transfer the chicken to a plate and shred it with a fork. Return it to the slow cooker, and cook on low for 30 minutes more before serving, allowing the chicken to absorb some of the liquid.
Nutrition: Per Serving (4 ounces): Calories: 188; Total fat: 3g; Protein: 22g; Carbs: 16g; Fiber: 0g; Sugar: 10g; Sodium: 7mg

Vegan Recipes

Fresh Tomato And Celery Soup

Servings: 4
Cooking Time: 30 Minutes
Ingredients:
- 1 lb. tomatoes, peeled, roughly chopped
- 4 oz celery root, finely chopped
- ¼ cup fresh celery leaves, finely chopped
- 1 tbsp fresh basil, finely chopped
- Salt and pepper
- 5 tbsp extra virgin olive oil

Directions:
1. Preheat the oil in a large non-stick frying pan over a medium-high temperature.
2. Add finely chopped celery root, celery leaves, and fresh basil. Season with salt and pepper and stir-fry for about 10 minutes, until nicely browned. Add chopped tomatoes and about ¼ cup of water. Reduce the heat to minimum and cook for 15 minutes, stirring constantly, until softened. Now add about 4 cups of water (or vegetable broth) and bring it to a boil. Give it a good stir and remove from the heat.
3. Top with fresh parsley and serve.

Nutrition:Per Serving: Net carbs 6.9 g; Fiber 1.9 g; Fats 10.8 g; Fatsr 2 g; Calories 122

Mini Vegetable Frittatas

Servings: 9
Cooking Time: 15 Minutes
Ingredients:
- 5 Eggs
- 2 ounces Goat cheese, shredded
- 2 tablespoons Low-fat milk
- 1 cup Tomato, chopped
- 2 cups Chopped broccoli, fresh
- ¼ teaspoon Pepper crushed
- ¼ teaspoon Salt
- Cooking spray

Directions:
1. Blend milk and eggs in a mixer bowl.
2. Add crumbled goat cheese and all the chopped vegetables in it and combine.
3. Season it with pepper and salt.
4. Spoon this mixture into muffin cups sprayed with cooking oil.
5. Bake it at 3°F for about 12-15 minutes until it becomes golden color on the top.
6. Serve hot.

Nutrition:Per Serving: Net carbs 3.9 g; Fiber 1.4 g; Fats 4.03 g; Fatsr 1 g; Calories .3

Butternut Squash And Black Bean Enchiladas

Servings: 8 Enchiladas
Cooking Time: 40 Minutes
Ingredients:
- 1 teaspoon extra-virgin olive oil
- 2 teaspoons minced garlic
- 1 onion, diced
- 1 jalapeño pepper, seeded and finely diced
- 1 red bell pepper, finely diced
- 1 small butternut squash (about 2½ pounds), peeled, seeds removed, and diced
- 1 teaspoon low-sodium taco seasoning
- 1 teaspoon ground cumin
- 1 (10-ounce) can diced tomatoes or 2 large fresh tomatoes, diced
- 1 (15.5-ounce) can black beans, drained and rinsed
- ¼ cup water
- 1 (10-ounce) can red enchilada sauce or about 1 cup Homemade Enchilada Sauce, divided
- 8 small whole-wheat tortillas, such as La Tortilla Factory low-carb tortillas
- 1 cup shredded Monterey Jack cheese
- ½ cup sliced black olives
- 2 scallions, chopped
- Post-Op
- 1 enchilada

Directions:
1. Preheat the oven to 425°F.
2. Place a large skillet (large enough to accommodate all the squash) over medium-high heat. Heat the olive oil and garlic for about 1 minute, or until the garlic is fragrant. Add the onion, jalapeño, and bell pepper. Sauté for 2 to 3 minutes, or until tender.
3. Add the squash, taco seasoning, and cumin. Sauté and stir for 2 minutes, until the seasonings are mixed well. Add the tomatoes, beans, and water. Cover the skillet and cook for 30 minutes, or until squash is tender.
4. Spread ¼ cup of enchilada sauce on the bottom of a 9-by-13-inch baking dish.
5. Place the tortillas on a clean work surface. Fill each tortilla with about ½ cup of the squash mixture. (There may be some left over.) Fold over each tortilla and place them seam-side down in the baking dish.
6. Pour the remaining (about ¾ cup) enchilada sauce over the top of the enchiladas. Top with the cheese. Cover with aluminum foil.
7. Bake for about 10 minutes, or until cheese is melted.
8. Garnish with the olives and scallions before serving.

Nutrition: Per Serving (1 enchilada): Calories: 233; Total fat: 8g; Protein: 13g; Carbs: 27g; Fiber: 6g; Sugar: 4g; Sodium: 6mg

Avocado Pineapple Salad

Servings: 3
Cooking Time: 20 Minutes
Ingredients:
- 1 cup avocado chunks
- 1 cup pineapple chunks
- 1 cup watermelon
- 1 cup sour cream
- 1 cup spinach, finely chopped
- 1 tbsp honey
- 1 tsp vanilla extract
- 1 tbsp flaxseeds

Directions:
1. In a medium bowl, combine sour cream, honey, vanilla extract, and flaxseeds. Stir well to combine and set aside.
2. Wash and prepare the vegetables.
3. Peel the avocado and pineapple and cut in half. Remove the pit from the avocado and cut into small chunks along with pineapple. Place in a large salad bowl and set aside.
4. Cut one large watermelon wedge and peel it. Cut into bite-sized pieces and discard the seeds. Add it to the bowl with other fruits and set aside.
5. Wash the spinach thoroughly under cold running water and roughly chop it. Add it to the bowl with other fruits.
6. Now, pour the sour cream mixture over the fruits and veggies and toss well to coat all the ingredients.
7. Refrigerate for 15 minutes before serving.
Nutrition:Per Serving: Net carbs 26.3 g;Fiber 5.g;Fats 25.9 g;Fatsr 2 g;Calories 343

Mini Eggplant Pizzas

Servings: 4
Cooking Time: 12 Minutes
Ingredients:
- 1 eggplant
- ¼ cup, pasta sauce
- 4 teaspoons, olive oil
- ½ teaspoon, salt
- 1/8 teaspoon, ground black pepper
- ½ cup, shredded part-skim mozzarella cheese
- Cooking spray
- Baking sheet

Directions:
1. Peel eggplant and cut into 4 half-inch-thick slices.
2. Preheat your toaster at 4°f.
3. Brush both parts of the eggplant with some cooking spray oil and season it with pepper and salt.
4. Arrange the pizza on a baking sheet and bake for 8 minutes, until it becomes browned and tender.
5. Flip sides and bake further 6 - 8 minutes.
6. Spread 1 tbsp of pasta sauce on all side of the sliced eggplant.
7. Top it with the shredded cheese.
8. Bake the cheese until it starts to melt for about 3 - 5 minutes.
9. Serve the dish hot.
Nutrition: Net carbs 8.9 g Fiber 3.2 g Fats 7.5 g Sugar 8 g Calories 119.1

Roasted Vegetable Quinoa Salad With Chickpeas

Servings:6
Cooking Time: 30 Minutes
Ingredients:
- 1 small eggplant, diced
- 1 small zucchini, diced
- 1 small yellow summer squash, diced
- ½ cup grape tomatoes, halved
- 1 (15-ounce) can chickpeas, drained and rinsed
- 3 tablespoons extra-virgin olive oil, divided
- ⅓ cup packaged quinoa
- 1 cup low-sodium vegetable or chicken broth
- 2 tablespoons freshly squeezed lemon juice
- 1 teaspoon minced fresh garlic or 1 garlic clove, minced
- 1 tablespoon dried basil
- 1 teaspoon dried oregano
- Post-Op
- ½ cup serving

Directions:
1. Preheat the oven to 425°F. Line a 9-by-13-inch baking sheet with parchment paper.
2. Spread the eggplant, zucchini, yellow squash, tomatoes, and chickpeas across the baking sheet and toss them with 1 tablespoon of olive oil.
3. Bake for 30 minutes, stirring once halfway through. The finished vegetables should be tender and the tomatoes should be juicy. The chickpeas will be firm and crispy.
4. While the vegetables and chickpeas are roasting, place the quinoa and broth in a small saucepan over medium-high heat. Cover and bring to a boil. Reduce the heat to low and cook for about 15 minutes, or until all liquid has absorbed. Remove the pan from the heat and fluff the quinoa with a fork. (Otherwise, make the quinoa according to the package instructions.)
5. In a small dish, whisk together the lemon juice, garlic, and remaining 2 tablespoons of olive oil. Mix in the basil and oregano.
6. In a large serving bowl, combine the quinoa, roasted vegetables with chickpeas, and dressing. Gently stir to combine. Serve and enjoy!
Nutrition: Per Serving (½ cup): Calories: 200; Total fat: 9g; Protein: ; Carbs: 27g; Fiber: 8g; Sugar: 4g; Sodium: 160mg

Blue Oatmeal Porridge

Servings: 2
Cooking Time: 5 Minutes
Ingredients:
- 1 cup, whole grain oatmeal
- 2 tablespoons, flaxseed meal, ground flax
- ½ tablespoon, dry cocoa powder, unsweetened
- 2 teaspoon, brown sugar
- ½ cup, blueberries, frozen, unsweetened
- 1½ cup, water

Directions:
1. Boil water in a pan.
2. Combine all of the dry ingredients in a mixing bowl and add to the boiling water.
3. Reduce the temperature and cook it for a couple of minutes as far as you get the desired consistency.
4. Top it with blueberries at the time of serving.
Nutrition: Net carbs 38.4 g Fiber 7 g Fats 7 g Sugar 1 g Calories 214.2

Oven-roasted Brussels Sprouts

Servings: 4
Cooking Time: 30 Minutes
Ingredients:
- 15 to 20, fresh brussels sprouts
- Non-fat spray for cooking
- 2 tablespoons, olive oil
- ½ teaspoon, ground black pepper
- ¼ teaspoon, salt

Directions:
1. Set your oven at 425°f and put it on for preheating.
2. Trim all the stems from sprouts.
3. Cut sprouts in lengthwise into wo equal parts.
4. Take a shallow baking dish and spray with cooking oil.
5. Place all the sprouts in the center of dish keep the cut-side up.
6. Drizzle olive oil on top of it.
7. Similarly, drizzle salt and ground pepper.
8. Bake it for 15 minutes, and flip sides after ten minutes.
9. Serve hot with fresh tomato soup or parmesan zucchini.

Nutrition: Net carbs 6.7 g Fiber 2.8 g Fats 3.6 g Sugar 2 g Calories 61.8

Garlic And Olive Oil Spaghetti Squash

Servings: 2
Cooking Time: 1 Hour
Ingredients:
- 1 spaghetti squash
- 2 tablespoons, olive oil
- 3 cloves garlic, minced
- ¼ cup water
- ¼ teaspoon, pepper crushed
- ¼ teaspoon, salt

Directions:
1. Cut the squash in lengthwise into two parts.
2. Scoop out all the seeds, and save the seeds.
3. In a casserole place the squash, face down and pour a quarter cup of water.
4. Bake the squash at 375°f temperature for 30 minutes.
5. Flip the squash to cook the other side for an extra 30 minutes until it becomes soft.
6. Allow squash to settle down.
7. Now, in a sauté pan pour olive oil and bring to low-medium heat.
8. When the oil becomes hot add garlic and sauté.
9. With the use of a serving fork, transfer the boiled squash into the sautéing pan. Add some salt and pepper.
10. Cook it for 3-5 minutes more.
11. Serve hot

Nutrition: Net carbs 14.5 g Fiber 2.9 g Fats 14.5 g Sugar 4 g Calories 181.4

Coconut Curry Tofu Bowl

Servings:6
Cooking Time: 30 Minutes
Ingredients:
- 1 (14-ounce) package extra-firm tofu
- 3 teaspoons coconut oil, divided
- 4 teaspoons minced garlic
- 1 tablespoon grated ginger
- 1 jalapeño pepper, seeds removed and finely diced
- 1 yellow or orange bell pepper, chopped
- 2 carrots, cut into ½-inch chunks
- 1 medium bok choy, stems cut into ½-inch pieces, leaves diced
- 2 tablespoons curry powder
- ½ teaspoon turmeric
- ½ teaspoon ground cumin
- ⅛ teaspoon ground cinnamon
- 2 cups unflavored, unsweetened coconut milk
- 4 ounces canned tomato sauce
- ½ cup low-sodium vegetable or chicken broth
- Cauliflower Rice
- ¼ cup chopped fresh cilantro, for garnish
- Post-Op
- ½ to 1 cup serving

Directions:
1. Drain the tofu and place it on a paper towel–lined plate or bowl. Cover with several layers of paper towel or a clean dish towel, and set a sauté pan on top for added weight. Let the tofu sit for 30 minutes to drain some of its excess water.
2. Place the tofu on a clean cutting board. Halve it lengthwise, and then cut into 1-by-2-inch cubes.
3. In a large nonstick pan over medium heat, heat 1½ teaspoons of coconut oil.
4. When the oil is very hot, add the tofu cubes and cook until lightly browned on all sides, 10 to 15 minutes. Transfer the tofu to a bowl and set aside.
5. In the same pan over medium heat, add the remaining 1½ teaspoons of coconut oil. Once the oil is very hot, add the garlic, ginger, jalapeño, bell pepper, carrots, and bok choy stems. Sauté for 10 minutes, or until the vegetables are crisp tender.
6. Add the curry powder, turmeric, cumin, and cinnamon and stir to coat.
7. Next, mix in the coconut milk, tomato sauce, and broth. Stir until smooth.
8. Gently mix in the tofu and bok choy leaves. Stir to coat and allow to simmer for 5 to 10 minutes, or until the leaves are wilted.
9. Prepare the bowls by layering the Cauliflower Rice and curry tofu vegetable mixture. Garnish each bowl with the cilantro.

Nutrition: Per Serving (1 cup): Calories: 219; Total fat: 8g; Protein: 15g; Carbs: 24g; Fiber: 11g; Sugar: ; Sodium: 337mg

Grilled Cheese Pizza Sandwich

Servings: 1
Cooking Time: 5 Minutes
Ingredients:
- 2 slices, multi-grain bread
- 2 tablespoons, marinara sauce
- 1 teaspoon, shredded parmesan
- ¼ cup, mozzarella cheese
- ¼ teaspoon, pepper ground
- ¼ teaspoon, salt

Directions:
1. Spread the marinara sauce on one side of both bread slice.
2. Now spread mozzarella cheese on top of one slice bread.
3. Sprinkle grated parmesan cheese on the top of the mozzarella.
4. Top it with 2nd piece of bread, keeping the sauce side down.
5. Now place it on a heated pan until the cheese starts to melt and the outer side becomes golden brown.
6. Serve hot.

Nutrition: Net carbs 26.3 g Fiber 4.4 g Fats 8.3 g Sugar 6 g Calories 242.3

Vegan Lentil Burgers

Servings: 8
Cooking Time: 1 Hour
Ingredients:
- 1 cup, brown rice, uncooked
- 1 cup, lentils, uncooked
- 1½ cup, carrots, finely grated
- 1½ cup, oatmeal, uncooked
- ½ teaspoon, garlic powder
- 1 teaspoon, salt
- 1 small onion, coarsely chopped
- 4 cups, water
- Cooking spray

Directions:
1. In a large bowl pour four cups of water and cook the rice and the lentils, at low heat for 45 minutes by keeping the lid closed.
2. After cooking, allow it to settle and cool.
3. Add all the remaining ingredients gradually and mix well.
4. Mold into patties
5. Spray some cooking oil and bring to low heart.
6. When the pan becomes hot, place the patties and cook for minutes until it becomes brown.
7. Flip sides and cook another 6 minutes.
8. Use as a burger with your favorite sauce.

Nutrition: Net carbs 24.2 g Fiber 4.8 g Fats 1.5 g Sugar 5 g Calories 127.6

Portobello Mushrooms Bake

Servings: 4
Cooking Time: 25 Minutes
Ingredients:
- 3 caps, portabella mushroom, large
- 2 cups, instant brown rice
- 1 cup, black bans
- 1 cup, red pepper pieces
- 2 tablespoons, olive oil
- 3 ounces, shredded mozzarella, part-skim
- ¼ teaspoon, garlic, minced
- ¼ teaspoon, salt

Directions:
1. In a medium saucepan pour olive oil and sauté red pepper and garlic until it becomes soft.
2. Add the mushrooms and continue sautéing for 5 minutes.
3. After cooking, stop heating and remove from the pan.
4. Now boil rice as per the given directions in the packet.
5. Mix the rice with black beans in a casserole dish.
6. Add the mushroom caps in the rice and black bean mix.
7. Make the topping with roasted red peppers and mozzarella cheese.
8. Bake at 350°f temperature for 20 minutes until cheese becomes bubbly.

Nutrition: Net carbs 3g Fiber 7.1 g Fats 10.5 g Sugar 5 g Calories 288.8

Spaghetti Squash Marinara

Servings: 2
Cooking Time: 50 Minutes
Ingredients:
- 1 raw spaghetti squash, medium
- 14 ½ ounces stewed tomatoes, cut up, canned
- 1 teaspoon, Italian seasoning
- 1 teaspoon, olive oil
- 1, small onion, chopped
- 1 teaspoon, garlic clove, minced
- ¼ cup, parmesan cheese, grated

Directions:
1. Set the oven at 350°f and start preheating.
2. Cut the squash lengthwise into two equal parts and scoop out all the seeds.
3. Place all the squash, in a large baking dish keeping the cut sides down and pierce the skin with a fork.
4. Bake it until it becomes soft for about 30 - minutes.
5. Now let us make the sauce.
6. Heat some oil in a small skillet on medium temperature.
7. Add garlic, onion and sauté about 5 minutes, until it becomes tender.
8. Add Italian seasoning, tomatoes and bring to boil.
9. Reduce the heat and continue cooking for about 5 minutes, without covering the skillet, until you get the desired consistency.
10. Now before serving, carefully take out the squash pulp in strands with a fork, as if looks like spaghetti.
11. Pour sauce on the top of the squash and sprinkle some parmesan cheese on top.

Nutrition: Net carbs 4 g Fiber 2.1 g Fats 3.3 g Sugar 1 g Calories 88.6

Red Lentil Soup With Kale

Servings:6
Cooking Time: 45 Minutes
Ingredients:
- 1 tablespoon extra-virgin olive oil
- 1 cup chopped onion
- ½ cup carrots, cut into ½-inch chunks
- ½ cup celery, cut into ¼-inch chunks
- 1 teaspoon minced garlic
- 1 cup red lentils
- 1 teaspoon dried thyme
- 1 teaspoon ground cumin
- 2 cups low-sodium vegetable broth
- 2 cups water
- 2 large stalks kale, stemmed, with leaves chopped (about 2 cups)
- 1 bay leaf
- 2 tablespoons freshly squeezed lemon juice
- Low-fat plain Greek yogurt (optional)
- Post-Op
- ¼ cup
- ½ cup
- 1 to 2 cups

Directions:
1. In a large stock pot over medium heat, heat the olive oil. Add the onion, carrots, celery, and garlic, and sauté until tender, 5 to 7 minutes.
2. Add the lentils, thyme, and cumin. Mix well and stir for 1 to 2 minutes, until all the ingredients are coated well with the seasonings.
3. Add the broth and water to the pot. Bring to a simmer, add the kale, and stir well. Add the bay leaf, then cover the pot and simmer for 30 to 35 minutes.
4. Remove the pot from the heat. Remove and discard the bay leaf. Stir in the lemon juice. Use an immersion blender to puree the soup to your desired consistency. Alternatively, let the soup cool for 10 minutes before pureeing it in batches in a blender.
5. Garnish each bowl of soup with a dollop of the Greek yogurt (if using) and serve.
Nutrition: Per Serving (1 cup): Calories: 170; Total fat: 3g; Protein: 13g; Carbs: 24g; Fiber: 3g; Sugar: 4g; Sodium: 59mg

Curried Eggplant And Chickpea Quinoa

Servings:8
Cooking Time: 20 Minutes
Ingredients:
- 4 teaspoons minced garlic
- 1 teaspoon extra-virgin olive oil
- 1 large onion, chopped
- 1 red bell pepper, chopped
- 1 tablespoon ground cumin
- 1 teaspoon ground turmeric
- 2 teaspoons smoked paprika
- ¼ teaspoon cayenne pepper
- ½ cup water
- 1 medium eggplant, cut into ½-inch chunks
- 1 yellow summer squash, cut into ½-inch chunks
- 3 tomatoes, diced
- 1 (15-ounce) can chickpeas, drained and rinsed
- ½ cup packaged quinoa
- 1 cup vegetable or chicken broth
- Low-fat plain Greek yogurt, for garnish
- Post-Op
- 1 cup

Directions:
1. Place a large skillet over medium-high heat. Sauté the garlic in the olive oil for 1 minute. Add the onion and bell pepper and sauté for 2 to 3 minutes, or until tender.
2. Stir in the cumin, turmeric, paprika, and cayenne pepper and cook for 1 to 2 minutes.
3. Add the water, eggplant, squash, tomatoes, and chickpeas. Cover, reduce the heat to medium-low, and cook for 15 minutes.
4. While the vegetables and chickpeas cook, place the quinoa and broth in a small saucepan over medium-high heat. Cover and bring to a boil. Reduce the heat to low and cook for about 15 minutes, or until all liquid has absorbed. Remove the pan from the heat and fluff the quinoa with a fork. (Otherwise, make the quinoa according to the package instructions.)
5. Serve the curried vegetables over the quinoa, garnished with a dollop of the yogurt.
Nutrition: Per Serving (1 cup): Calories: 131; Total fat: 2g; Protein: ; Carbs: 23g; Fiber: 6g; Sugar: 6g; Sodium: 127mg

Barley-mushroom Risotto

Servings:6
Cooking Time: 55 Minutes
Ingredients:
- 1 tablespoon extra-virgin olive oil
- 1 teaspoon minced garlic
- 2 leeks, cleaned, ends removed and finely chopped, both white and green parts
- 4 cups sliced mushrooms
- 2 teaspoons dried thyme
- ½ cup pearl barley
- ½ cup dry white wine
- 1½ cups low-sodium vegetable or chicken broth
- 1 cup water
- 3 cups fresh spinach leaves
- Post-Op
- ½ cup

Directions:
1. Place a large skillet over medium heat. Sauté the olive oil and garlic for 1 minute. Add the leeks and sauté for 2 to 3 minutes, or until tender.
2. Add the mushrooms and cook until tender and browned, about 4 minutes.
3. Stir in the thyme and barley. Cook for another 2 minutes.
4. Add the wine and stir. Simmer for about 5 minutes, or until the liquid is absorbed.
5. Add the broth and water. Reduce the heat to low, cover the skillet, and simmer for 40 minutes. Stir occasionally to make sure the barley does not stick to the bottom of the pan.
6. Gently stir in the spinach and mix until it is wilted. Serve immediately.
Nutrition: Per Serving (½ cup): Calories: 104; Total fat: 3g; Protein: 3g; Carbs: 16g; Fiber: 3g; Sugar: 1g; Sodium: 40mg

Eggplant Rollatini

Servings:6 To 8 Rollatini
Cooking Time: 50 Minutes
Ingredients:
- Nonstick cooking spray
- 1 large eggplant
- 1 tablespoon salt
- 1 teaspoon extra-virgin olive oil
- 1 pound fresh spinach (about 10 cups)
- ½ cup part-skim ricotta cheese
- ¾ cup shredded part-skim mozzarella cheese, divided
- ¼ cup shredded Parmigiano-Reggiano cheese
- 1 egg
- 1 teaspoon minced garlic
- ½ cup Marinara Sauce with Italian Herbs or low-sugar jarred marinara sauce, divided
- Post-Op
- 2 rollatinis

Directions:
1. Preheat the oven to 400°F. Spray 1 or 2 baking sheets with the cooking spray.
2. Slice the eggplant lengthwise into ¼-inch pieces. Lay the slices on a paper towel and sprinkle them with salt. Let them sit for 10 minutes to help release some of the water in the eggplant. Pat dry afterward. It's okay to wipe off some of the salt before baking.
3. Place the eggplant on the baking sheet and bake for 10 minutes. Remove from the oven and set aside to cool. Leave the oven on.
4. Put a large pot over medium-high heat. Heat the olive oil for 1 minute. Add the spinach leaves and cook, stirring occasionally, for about 3 minutes or until wilted. Set aside to let cool.
5. Combine the ricotta, ¼ cup of mozzarella, Parmigiano-Reggiano, egg, and garlic in a medium bowl. Mix well. When the spinach is cool, gently stir it into the cheese mixture.
6. Spread ¼ cup of the marinara sauce across the bottom of an 8-by-8-inch baking dish.
7. Spread the cheese mixture (about 2 tablespoons each) onto each eggplant slice, roll the slice, and place seam-side down in the baking dish. Continue until all eggplant slices are made into roll-ups and placed in the pan.
8. Top the rolled eggplant with the remaining ¼ cup of marinara and ½ cup of mozzarella.
9. Reduce the oven temperature to 350°F. Cover the baking sheets with aluminum foil and bake for 30 minutes. Remove the foil and bake for an additional 10 minutes, or until the cheese is brown and bubbly.

Nutrition: Per Serving (2 rollatini): Calories: 160; Total fat: 7g; Protein: 11g; Carbs: 16g; Fiber: 6g; Sugar: 8g; Sodium: 330mg

Mexican Stuffed Summer Squash

Servings:2
Cooking Time: 33 Minutes
Ingredients:
- Nonstick cooking spray
- 1 yellow summer squash
- ½ cup Refried Black Beans or canned fat-free refried pinto beans with 1 teaspoon taco seasoning mixed in (for flavor)
- ½ cup cooked quinoa
- ¼ cup shredded Colby Jack cheese
- 1 small tomato, diced
- 2 tablespoons sliced black olives
- 2 scallions, chopped, for garnish
- Post-Op
- 1 stuffed squash half

Directions:
1. Preheat the oven to 400°F. Coat an 8-by-8-inch baking dish with the cooking spray.
2. Cut the ends off of the summer squash and discard. Cut lengthwise, then use a spoon to remove and discard the seeds. Place the squash halves cut-side down in the baking dish. Gently poke a couple of holes in the squash to vent. Add 1 tablespoon of water to the dish. Microwave for about 3 minutes or until slightly tender. Discard any leftover water.
3. When cool enough to handle, turn the squash so they are skin-side down and spaced evenly apart in the dish.
4. Layer ¼ cup of the beans in each squash, then ¼ cup of the quinoa. Top the whole thing with the Colby Jack cheese. Cover with aluminum foil and bake for 25 minutes. Remove the foil and bake for 5 minutes more, or until the cheese is bubbly and the squash is tender.
5. Garnish each squash with the tomatoes, olives, and scallions just before serving.

Nutrition: Per Serving (1 squash half): Calories: 190; Total fat: 8 g; Protein: 9g; Carbs: 21g; Fiber: 4g; Sugar: 3g; Sodium: 40mg

Soup Recipes

Vegan Winter Lentil Stew

Servings: 8
Cooking Time: 50 Minutes
Ingredients:
- 2 - tbsp olive oil
- 1 - yellow onion
- 4 - cloves garlic
- 4 - carrots (about 1/2 lb.)
- 4 - stalks celery
- 2 - lbs. potatoes
- 1 - cup brown lentils
- 1 - tsp dried rosemary
- ½ - tsp dried thyme
- 2 - tbsp dijon mustard
- 1.5 - tbsp soy sauce
- 1 - tbsp brown sugar
- 6 - cups vegetable broth
- 1 - cup frozen peas

Directions:
1. Bones the onion and mince the garlic. Include the olive oil, onion, and garlic to a huge soup pot and start to sauté over medium warmth.
2. While the onion and garlic are sautéing, dice the celery, at that point add it to the pot and keep on sauté. As the celery, onion, and garlic are sautéing, strip and hack the carrots into half adjusts.
3. Add the carrots to the pot and keep on sauté.
4. Quickly mix the fixings to join, at that point placeBeef, Mushroom and Barley Soup a cover on the pot, turn the warmth up to high, and heat the stew up to the point of boiling.
5. When it arrives at a bubble, turn the warmth down to low and give it a chance to stew for 30mints, blending once in a while.
6. Close to the part of the bargain, when the potatoes are delicate, start to squash the potatoes a piece as you mix. This will help thicken the stew.
7. At last, following 30 minutes, blend in the solidified peas and enable them to warm through.
8. Taste the stew and include salt if necessary (This will rely upon the salt substance of your soup, I didn't include any extra).
9. Serve hot and appreciate!
Nutrition: Calories: 213 Carbs: 41g Fat: 5g Protein: 9g

Cauliflower And Sweet Corn Bisque

Servings: 4
Cooking Time: 50 Minutes
Ingredients:
- 2 to 3 - tablespoons extra-virgin olive oil
- 1 - large onion, chopped
- 1 - small-medium-sized head of cauliflower, chopped
- 2 - cloves garlic, chopped
- 2 - ears sweet corn
- Salt to taste
- White pepper to taste
- Pinch of cayenne pepper
- 1 - tablespoon butter
- Fresh thyme or other fresh herbs for garnish

Directions:
1. Warm the olive oil in a substantial bottomed pot. Include the onions and a spot of salt and cook on low heat, blending once in a while, for 5mints or until translucent.
2. Include the hacked cauliflower and garlic and increment warmth to medium. Include another spot of salt alongside white pepper and discretionary cayenne pepper. Cook, blending sometimes until cauliflower is delicately brilliant sautéed and marginally relaxed about 5mints.
3. In the meantime, shuck the corn and cut the pieces from both. Put a large portion of the bits in a safe spot, and add the rest of the parts to the pot alongside both of the cobs. Add simply enough water to cover the ears and heat blend to the point of boiling, mixing at times. Diminish to a stew and let cook for mints.
4. Take off the corn cobs from the soup. Utilizing a hand blender, puree the soup altogether. Add the saved corn parts to the soup and cook a couple of minutes to warm through. Add salt and pepper to taste, and blend in the discretionary spread. Present with the discretionary crisp herbs for trimming.
Nutrition: Calories: 200 carbs: 17g fat: 13g protein: 6g

Chunky Beef, Cabbage, And Tomato Soup

Servings: 7
Cooking Time: 30 Minutes
Ingredients:
- 1 - lb. 90% lean ground beef
- 1 ½ - teaspoon kosher salt
- ½ - cup diced onion
- ½ - cup diced celery
- ½ - cup diced carrot
- 28 - oz can diced or crushed tomatoes
- 5 - cups chopped green cabbage
- 4 - cups beef stock, canned* or homemade
- 2 - bay leaves

Directions:
1. Instant pot:
2. Expecting your electric weight cooker has a sauté choice, or if utilizing the instant pot, press the sauté catch and let the weight cooker gets hot, when hot shower with oil, include the ground hamburger and salt and cook until sautéed separating the meat into little pieces as it cooks, 3 to 4mints.
3. Whenever seared, include the onion, celery, and carrots and sauté 4 to 5mints.
4. Include the tomatoes, cabbage, meat stock, and inlet leaves, lock the cover cook high-weight 20mints.
5. Give the steam a chance to discharge normally. Expel cove leaves and serve. Makes 11cups.
6. Stove top:
7. Pursue indistinguishable headings from above in a huge pot or Dutch stove, cook secured low 40mints.
Nutrition: Calories: 1 Carbo: 14g, Protein: 15.5g, Fat: 6g, Sugar: 4.5g.

Chicken Soup With Spinach And Whole Wheat Acini Di Pepe

Servings: 4
Cooking Time: 25 Minutes
Ingredients:
- 4 - boneless skinless chicken thighs,
- ¼ - teaspoon kosher salt
- 1 - teaspoon olive oil
- ½ - cup diced onion
- ½ - cup diced celery
- ½ - cup peeled and sliced carrot
- 3 - cloves garlic, minced
- 4 - cups low-sodium chicken broth
- 2 - bay leaves
- Black pepper, to taste
- 2 - cups baby spinach
- ½ - cup delallo whole wheat acini di pepe, 2.5 oz

Directions:
1. Season the chicken with salt.
2. Warm the oil in a medium nonstick pot over medium warmth. Include the onion, celery, carrot, and garlic and sauté until delicate, 4 to 5mints.
3. Include the chicken, stock, inlet leaves, and 1/8 teaspoon dark pepper and heat to the point of boiling. Spread and lessen to medium-low until the chicken shreds effectively, around 25mints.
4. Dispose of the cove leaves, coarsely shred the chicken with two forks and come back to the soup, including the pasta and cook as indicated by bundle bearings, including the child spinach at last to wither.
Nutrition: Calories: 266, carb: 2, protein: 28g, fat: 6g, sugar: 3g.

Matzo Ball Soup

Servings: 5
Cooking Time: 1hr 30 Minutes
Ingredients:

* Soup:
* 1 - tbsp vegetable
* 2 - cloves garlic
* 1 - yellow onion
* 3 - carrots
* 3 - stalks celery
* 1 - chicken breast
* 6 - cups chicken broth
* 2 - cups of water
* Freshly cracked pepper
* Few sprigs fresh dill
* Matzo balls:
* 3 - large eggs
* 3 - tbsp vegetable or canola oil
* ¾ - cup matzo meal
* 1 - tsp salt
* ½ - tsp baking powder
* Freshly cracked pepper
* 3 - tbsp water

Directions:

1. Mince the garlic and bones the onion, celery, and carrots. Sauté the garlic, onion, celery, and carrots with the vegetable oil in an enormous pot over medium warmth until the onions are delicate and straightforward.
2. Include the chicken bosom, chicken stock, cups water, some crisply split pepper, and a couple of sprigs of dill to the pot. Spot a cover on the pot and let it come up to a bubble. When it arrives at a bubble, turn the warmth down to low and give it a chance to stew for 30mints.
3. While the soup is stewing, blend the matzo ball mixture. In a medium bowl, whisk together the eggs and vegetable oil. Include the matzo dinner, salt, heating powder, and a little newly split pepper to the eggs and oil. Blend until all-around joined. At last, include tbsp water and blend until smooth once more. Refrigerate the blend for 30mints to permit the matzo supper time to retain the dampness.
4. After the chicken soup has stewed, cautiously take off the chicken bosom and shred it with a fork.

Return the destroyed chicken to the soup. Taste the stock and change the salt if necessary.
5. When the matzo ball combination has refrigerated and hardened up, start to frame it into ping pong estimated balls. Drop the balls into the stewing soup as they're fashioned, restoring the top to the pot after everyone. When all of the matzo balls are within the soup, let them stew for 20mints without evacuating the quilt. Ensure the soup is delicately stewing the complete time.
6. Include a few sprigs of crisp dill simply earlier than serving.

Nutrition: Calories: 120 Carbs: 15g Fat: 5g Protein: 3g

Beef, Mushroom And Barley Soup

Servings: 3
Cooking Time: 1hr 15minutes
Ingredients:

* 1 - lb. Beef cubes, cut from a chuck roast.
* ¼ - red onion, chopped
* 2 - garlic cloves, crushed
* 1 15 - oz can mushroom, drained
* 2 - cups homemade beef broth
* 2.5 - cups water
* ½ - cup pearled barley
* Salt and pepper to taste
* Fresh parsley to garnish (optional)
* Homemade bread from the freezer
* 15 - oz. Can corn

Directions:

1. Dark-colored the perimeters of the beef 3-d shapes in a good-sized pan with the crimson onion and squashed garlic.
2. When all facets have sautéed, consist of the hamburger inventory and water.
3. Heat to the factor of boiling, at that point, include the pearled grain.
4. Let cook at a shifting bubble for 20mints.
5. Season with salt and pepper to flavor.
6. Get equipped rolls.
7. Warm corn as coordinated at the can.
8. Serve with bread and corn.

Nutrition: Calories: 1 Carbs: 23g Fat: 8g Protein: 9g

Fish and Seafood Recipes

Microwave Grilled Salmon

Servings: 4
Cooking Time: 4 Minutes
Ingredients:
- 1½ pound, Salmon
- 2 tablespoons, Olive oil
- 1 tablespoon, Lemon juice1 clove, Garlic, minced
- ¼ teaspoon, Salt¼ teaspoon, Ground pepper

Directions:
1. Set your microwave to grill cooking.
2. In a medium bowl, mix all the ingredients.
3. Marinate the salmon.
4. Grill the fish.
5. Serve hot.

Nutrition:Per Serving: Net carbs 0.4 g;Fiber 1 g;Fats 9.5 g;Fatsr 2 g;Calories 210.2

Slow-roasted Pesto Salmon

Servings:4
Cooking Time: 20 Minutes
Ingredients:
- 4 (6-ounce) salmon fillets
- 1 teaspoon extra-virgin olive oil
- 4 tablespoons Perfect Basil Pesto
- Post-Op
- 2 ounces
- 3 to 6 ounces

Directions:
1. Preheat the oven to 275°F. Line a rimmed baking sheet with aluminum foil and brush the foil with the olive oil.
2. Place the salmon fillets skin-side down on the baking sheet.
3. Spread 1 tablespoon of pesto on each fillet.
4. Roast the salmon for about 20 minutes, or just until opaque in the center.
5. Serve immediately.

Nutrition: Per Serving (3 ounces): Calories: 182; Total fat: 10g; Protein: 20g; Carbs: 1g; Fiber: 0g; Sugar: 0g; Sodium: 90mg

Marinated Tuna

Servings: 6
Cooking Time: 10 Minutes
Ingredients:
- 2 lbs. tuna steaks, boneless
- ¼ cup fresh coriander, chopped
- 2 garlic cloves, minced
- 2 tablespoons lemon juice
- 1 cup olive oil½ tsp smoked paprika
- ½ tsp cumin, ground
- ½ tsp chili pepper, ground
- ½ tsp salt
- ¼ tsp black pepper, ground

Directions:
1. Add the coriander, garlic, paprika, cumin, chili and lemon juice in a food processor and pulse to combine. Gradually add in the oil and mix the ingredients until a smooth mixture.
2. Transfer the mixture into a bowl, add the fish and gently toss to coat the fish evenly with sauce. Chill for at least hours to allow the flavors to penetrate into the fish.

3. Remove the fish from the chiller and preheat the grill. Lightly brush the grid with oil, place the fish on the grid, and grill for about to 4 minutes on each side.
4. Remove the fish from the grill, transfer to a serving plate and serve with lemon wedges or some vegetables.

Nutrition:Per Serving: Net carbs 0.7 g;Fiber 1 g;Fats 11.9 g;Fatsr 4 g;Calories 303

Seafood Cioppino

Servings:8
Cooking Time: 45 Minutes
Ingredients:
- 2 teaspoons minced garlic
- 1 tablespoon extra-virgin olive oil
- 2 leeks, washed and cut into ⅛-inch slices, both white and green parts
- 2 celery stalks, cut into ¼-inch pieces
- 1 green bell pepper, diced
- 4 cups water
- 1½ cups dry white wine
- 1 (10-ounce) container grape tomatoes
- 1 large tomato, chopped into ¼-inch pieces
- ½ teaspoon dried thyme
- ½ teaspoon dried basil
- 1 bay leaf
- 1 tablespoon chopped fresh parsley
- Juice of ½ lemon
- 2 pounds shrimp, deveined
- 1 (6-ounce) can lump crabmeat, drained and cartilage removed
- ½ pound scallops
- 1 teaspoon freshly ground black pepper
- Post-Op
- ½ cup
- 1 cup

Directions:
1. Place a large pot or Dutch oven over medium heat. Sauté the garlic in the olive oil for 1 to 2 minutes. Add the leeks and stir for about 2 minutes, or until tender.
2. Add the celery and green pepper and cook for about 5 minutes, or until tender.
3. Pour in the water, wine, tomatoes, thyme, basil, bay leaf, parsley, and lemon juice. Bring to a boil, then cover, reduce the heat to low, and let simmer for 25 minutes.
4. Remove and discard the bay leaf. Add the shrimp, crabmeat, and scallops. Bring back to a simmer and cook for 5 to 10 minutes, or until the shrimp are no longer pink and the scallops are opaque. Stir in the black pepper.
5. Ladle into soup bowls and serve.

Nutrition: Per Serving (1 cup): Calories: 171; Total fat: 4g; Protein: 21g; Carbs: 5g; Fiber: 0g; Sugar: 1g; Sodium: 4mg

Fried-less Friday Fish Fry With Cod

Servings:4
Cooking Time: 10 Minutes
Ingredients:
- ¾ cup corn meal
- ¾ cup whole-wheat bread crumbs
- 1½ teaspoons lemon pepper seasoning
- ½ teaspoon onion powder
- ½ teaspoon garlic powder
- ¼ teaspoon ground cayenne pepper
- 2 eggs
- 4 (4-ounce) cod fillets
- 1½ tablespoons extra-virgin olive oil
- Post-Op
- ¼ cup or 2 ounces pureed (try pureeing with Greek yogurt-based tartar sauce for flavor and consistency)
- 4 ounces

Directions:
1. Preheat oven to 450°F.
2. Combine cornmeal, bread crumbs, lemon pepper seasoning, onion powder, garlic powder, and cayenne pepper in a large resealable bag. Shake to mix and set aside.
3. In a small bowl, lightly beat the eggs.
4. Carefully add a fish fillet to the bag to coat it with the dry mixture. Next, dip it into the egg, then coat it a second time in the dry mixture. Set aside on a plate and repeat with the remaining fillets.
5. Place a large oven-safe skillet over medium heat. Add the oil and allow it to heat for 1 minute.
6. Carefully add the fish to the skillet. Brown it on one side for 2 minutes and then gently turn to brown the other side for another 2 minutes.
7. Transfer the skillet to the oven. Bake for 6 to 7 minutes, or until golden brown and flaky.
Nutrition: Per Serving (4-ounce fillet): Calories: 297; Total fat: 9g; Protein: 27g; Carbs: 2; Fiber: 3g; Sugar: 0g; Sodium: 576mg

Grilled Mediterranean Ahi Tuna

Servings: 4
Cooking Time: 10 Minutes
Ingredients:
- 4½ ounces, Ahi tuna steaks, Fresh
- 1 tablespoon, Extra virgin olive oil
- ½ teaspoon Salt½ teaspoon, Lemon juice
- ¼ teaspoon, Cracked black pepper
- ½ teaspoon, Oregano, finely chopped
- ¼ teaspoon, Red pepper, ground1 teaspoon, Basil, finely chopped
- 1 clove Garlic, finely minced

Directions:
1. Set the charcoal grill on high heat for 30 minutes before you start grilling the tuna steak.
2. Wash and clean the tuna.
3. Pat dry before marinating and put in a shallow bowl.
4. In a small bowl mix all the spices with oil and lemon juice.

5. Allow the mixture to have a rest for minutes so that everything blends well. If you are sensitive to spices, use a fork/spoon to mix the spices.
6. Now, marinate the tuna steaks applying the mixture with a brush.
7. Allow it to settle for 5 minutes.
8. Grill all the steaks on a hot grill at least for 3-5 minutes for both sides to get the desired result.
9. When the fish grilled well, it will turn to pinkish at the center.
10. Don't overcook.
Nutrition:Per Serving: Net carbs 0.5 g;Fiber 0.1 g;Fats 5.3 g;Fatsr 4 g;Calories 229.2

Baked Cod With Fennel And Kalamata Olives

Servings:4
Cooking Time: 35 Minutes
Ingredients:
- 2 teaspoons extra-virgin olive oil
- 1 fennel bulb, sliced paper thin
- ¼ cup dry white wine
- ⅛ cup freshly squeezed orange juice
- 1 teaspoon freshly ground black pepper
- 4 (4-ounce) cod fillets
- 4 slices fresh orange (with rind)
- ¼ cup Kalamata olives, pitted
- 2 bay leaves
- Post-Op
- 2 to 4 ounces
- 4 ounces

Directions:
1. Preheat the oven to 400°F.
2. Place a large Dutch oven or oven-safe skillet over medium heat and add the olive oil. Add the fennel and cook, stirring occasionally, until softened, 8 to 10 minutes.
3. Add the wine. Bring it to a simmer and cook for 1 to 2 minutes. Stir in the orange juice and pepper and simmer for 2 minutes more.
4. Remove the skillet from the heat and arrange the cod on top of the fennel mixture. Place the orange slices over the fillets. Position the olives and bay leaves around fish.
5. Roast for 20 minutes, or until fish is opaque. The fish is done when it flakes easily with a fork or reaches an internal temperature of 145°F. Remove the bay leaves prior to serving.
Nutrition: Per Serving (4 ounces): Calories: 18 Total fat: 5g; Protein: 21g; Carbs: 8g; Fiber: 3g; Sugar: 4g; Sodium: 271mg

Lemon-parsley Crab Cakes

Servings:4
Cooking Time: 10 Minutes
Ingredients:
- 3 tablespoons whole-wheat bread crumbs
- 1 egg, lightly beaten
- ½ teaspoon Dijon mustard
- 1½ tablespoons olive oil-based mayonnaise
- ¼ teaspoon ground cayenne pepper
- 2 teaspoons chopped fresh parsley
- Juice of ½ lemon
- 2 (6-ounce) cans lump crabmeat, drained and cartilage removed
- Nonstick cooking spray
- Post-Op
- ½ crab cake
- 1 crab cake

Directions:
1. In a medium bowl, mix together the bread crumbs, egg, mustard, mayonnaise, cayenne pepper, parsley, and lemon juice.
2. Very gently fold in the lump crabmeat.
3. Using a ¼-cup measuring cup, shape the mixture into 4 individual patties. Put the patties in the refrigerator and let sit for 30 minutes.
4. Preheat the oven to 500°F while the crab cakes rest in the refrigerator. Coat a baking sheet with the cooking spray.
5. Place the crab cakes on the baking sheet and bake on the center rack of the oven 10 minutes, or until starting to brown.
6. Serve immediately.
Nutrition: Per Serving (1 crab cake): Calories: 148; Total fat: 4g; Protein: 21g; Carbs: 5g; Fiber: 0g; Sugar: 1g; Sodium: 464mg

Grilled Lemon Shrimps

Servings: 3
Cooking Time: 6 Minutes
Ingredients:
- 1 lb. fresh shrimps, cleaned
- 1 tbsp fresh rosemary
- 4 tbsp extra-virgin olive oil
- 1 tsp garlic powder
- 2 tbsp lemon juice, freshly squeezed
- ½ tsp salt
- ½ tsp black pepper, freshly ground
- ½ tsp dried thyme, ground
- ½ tsp dried oregano, ground
- 1 organic lemon, sliced into wedges

Directions:
1. Combine olive oil, garlic, lemon juice, salt, pepper, thyme, and oregano in a medium bowl and mix until well incorporated. Place the shrimp and coat evenly with the marinade mixture. Cover the bowl and chill for at least hour to marinate the shrimps.
2. Preheat the grill to a medium-high temperature. Brush the grill grids with some oil.
3. Insert 2 to shrimps on each skewer, brush with marinade and grill for 3 minutes. Turn and grill the other side for another 3 minutes. Transfer to a serving platter.
4. Serve warm with lemons wedges and sprinkle with chopped parsley.
Nutrition: Per Serving:Net carbs 6.2 g;Fiber 2 g;Fats 21.6 g;Fatsr 3 g;Calories 3

Tuna Salad

Servings: 4

Cooking Time: 10 Minutes
Ingredients:
- 2 pounds, Tuna cooked
- 1 stalk, Celery, finely chopped
- 2/3 cup, Cottage cheese, non-fat
- 4 tablespoons, Plain yogurt, low-fat
- ¼, Small onion, red, coarsely chopped
- 1 teaspoon, Dijon mustard1 teaspoon, Lemon juice
- ¼ teaspoon, Dill
- ½ teaspoon, Salt

Directions:
1. In a large bowl, mix all the ingredients to make the salad.
2. Ideal for making sandwiches.
Nutrition:Per Serving: Net carbs 11.7 gFiber 0.6 g;Fats 2.2 g;Fatsr 1 g;Calories 190.3

Shrimp Cocktail Salad

Servings:4
Cooking Time: 5 Minutes
Ingredients:
- 1 lemon, halved and seeded
- 1 tablespoon black peppercorns
- 1 teaspoon dried thyme
- 1 bay leaf
- 1 pound unpeeled shrimp (31–35 count)
- ⅓ cup Seafood Sauce
- 3 tablespoons low-fat plain Greek yogurt
- ¼ cup olive oil-based mayonnaise
- 1 large head romaine lettuce, chopped
- ½ seedless cucumber, chopped
- Post-Op
- 4 shrimp pureed with 1 tablespoon Seafood Sauce (no lettuce or mayo-based dressing)
- 8 shrimp with ¼ head of lettuce and 3 tablespoons dressing

Directions:
1. Fill a large pot with water. Squeeze the juice from the lemon halves into the water, and add the black peppercorns, thyme, and bay leaf. Place the pot over high heat and bring to a boil.
2. While the water is heating, create an ice bath by filling a large bowl with ice and water. Set aside.
3. Add the shrimp to the boiling water and cook them for 2 to 3 minutes, or until they just turn pink.
4. Drain the shrimp in a colander and immediately put them in the ice bath to cool.
5. Once cool, peel the shrimp and remove the tails.
6. In a large bowl, combine the seafood sauce, yogurt, and mayonnaise. Mix well.
7. Add the cooked shrimp to the dressing and stir to coat.
8. Divide the lettuce among 4 plates. Add the cucumber and top it with the dressed shrimp.
9. Serve immediately.
Nutrition: Per Serving (8 shrimp with ¼ head of lettuce and 3 tablespoons dressing): Calories: 163; Total fat: 6g; Protein: 17g; Carbs: 4g; Fiber: 1g; Sugar: 4g; Sodium: 650mg

Tuna Noodle-less Casserole

Servings:10
Cooking Time: 40 Minutes
Ingredients:
- Nonstick cooking spray
- 1 medium red onion, chopped
- 1 red bell pepper, chopped
- 1½ cups diced tomato
- 3 cups fresh green beans
- ⅓ cup olive oil-based mayonnaise
- 1 (14.5-ounce) can condensed cream of mushroom soup
- ½ cup low-fat milk
- 1 cup shredded Cheddar cheese
- ½ teaspoon freshly ground black pepper
- 8 (5-ounce) cans water-packed albacore tuna, drained
- Post-Op
- ½ cup
- 1 cup

Directions:
1. Preheat the oven to 425°F.
2. Coat a large skillet with the cooking spray and place it over medium heat. Add the onion, red bell pepper, and tomatoes and sauté for about 5 minutes, or until the vegetables are tender and the tomatoes start to soften. Remove the skillet from the heat and set aside.
3. Cut off the stem ends of the green beans, and snap them into 3- to 4-inch pieces.
4. Fill a large saucepot ⅓ full with water, and place a steamer basket inside. Place the pot over high heat, and bring the water to a boil.
5. Add the green beans to the steamer basket, cover the pot, and reduce the heat to medium. Steam the green beans for 5 minutes. Immediately remove them from the heat, drain, and set aside.
6. Coat a 9-by-13-inch baking dish with the cooking spray.
7. In a large bowl, mix together the mayonnaise, condensed soup, milk, and cheese. Season the mixture with the black pepper.
8. Add the tuna, green beans, and sautéed vegetables to the bowl, and mix to combine. Pour the mixture into the baking dish.
9. Bake for 30 minutes, or until edges start to brown. Serve.

Nutrition: Per Serving (1 cup): Calories: 147; Total fat: 7g; Protein: 15g; Carbs: 6g; Fiber: 2g; Sugar: 2g; Sodium: 318mg

Broiled White Fish Parmesan

Servings: 4
Cooking Time: 10 Minutes
Ingredients:
- 3 ounces, Codfish
- ¼ cup, Parmesan cheese, grated
- 2 tablespoons, Light margarine, softened
- 1/8 teaspoon, Garlic salt
- 1/8 teaspoon, Ground black pepper
- 1 tablespoon, Lemon juice
- 1 tablespoon and 1½ teaspoons, Mayonnaise
- 1/8 teaspoon, Dried basil
- 1/8teaspoon, Onion powder
- Cooking spray

Directions:
1. Set the grill on high temperature and preheat before start cooking.
2. Grease the broiling pot with cooking spray.
3. Combine butter, Parmesan cheese, lemon juice and mayonnaise.
4. Season it with pepper, onion powder, dried basil, and garlic salt.
5. Mix it well and keep ready to use.
6. Layer the fillets on the broiler pan and broil for 2-3 minutes.
7. Flip it and cook for another 2-3 minutes.
8. Remove the baked fillets from the grill onto a plate and transfer the Parmesan mixture over it.
9. Again, broil it for a couple of minutes until the topping becomes brown.
10. Serve hot, when the flakes can easily remove.

Nutrition:Per Serving: Net carbs 1 g;Fiber 1 g;Fats 8.2 g;Fatsr 2 g;Calories 197.1 g

Wild Salmon Salad

Servings: 2
Cooking Time: 10 Minutes
Ingredients:
- 2 medium-sized cucumbers, sliced
- A handful of iceberg lettuce, torn¼ cup sweet corn
- 1 large tomato, roughly chopped
- 8 oz smoked wild salmon, sliced
- 4 tbsp freshly squeezed orange juice
- Dressing:
- 1 ¼ cup liquid yogurt, 2% fat
- 1 tbsp fresh mint, finely chopped
- 2 garlic cloves, crushed
- 1 tbsp sesame seeds

Directions:
1. Combine vegetables in a large bowl. Drizzle with orange juice and top with salmon slices. Set aside.
2. In another bowl, whisk together yogurt, mint, crushed garlic, and sesame seeds.
3. Drizzle over salad and toss to combine. Serve cold.

Nutrition:Per Serving: Net carbs 32.8 g;Fiber 3.2 g;Fats 11 g;Fatsr 2 g;Calories 2

Baked Halibut With Tomatoes And White Wine

Servings:6
Cooking Time: 35 Minutes
Ingredients:
- 3 tablespoons of extra-virgin olive oil
- 1 Vidalia onion, chopped
- 1 tablespoon minced garlic
- 1 (10-ounce) container grape tomatoes
- ¾ cup dry white wine, divided
- 3 tablespoons capers
- 1½ pounds thick-cut halibut fillet, deboned
- ½ teaspoon dried oregano
- Salt
- Freshly ground black pepper
- Post-Op
- 2 to 4 ounces
- 4 ounces

Directions:
1. Preheat the oven to 350°F.
2. In a Dutch oven or large oven-safe skillet over medium-high heat, heat the olive oil. Add the onion and sauté until browned and softened, 3 to 5 minutes.
3. Add the garlic and cook until fragrant, 1 to 2 minutes.
4. Add the tomatoes and cook for 5 minutes, or until they start to soften. Once the tomatoes start to soften, carefully use a potato masher to gently crush the tomatoes just enough to release their juices.
5. Add ½ cup of the wine to the pan and stir. Cook 2 to 3 minutes until slightly thickened. Stir in the capers.
6. Push the vegetables to the sides of the pan leaving the center of the pan open for the fish. Place the fish in the pan and sprinkle it with the oregano, salt, and pepper, then scoop the tomato mixture over the fish.
7. Pour in the remaining ¼ cup of wine.
8. Place in the oven and bake for about 20 minutes, uncovered, or until the fish flakes easily with a fork or reaches an internal temperature of 145°F. Serve.

Nutrition: Per Serving (4 ounces): Calories: 237; Total fat: 10g; Protein: 24g; Carbs: 6g; Fiber: 1g; Sugar: 2g; Sodium: 166mg

Slowly Roasted Pesto Salmon

Servings: 4
Cooking Time: 20 Minutes
Ingredients:
- 4 salmon fillets
- 1 teaspoon extra-virgin olive oil
- 4 tablespoons basil pesto

Directions:
1. Pre-heat your oven to 275 degrees F.
2. Line a rimmed baking sheet with foil and brush with olive oil.
3. Transfer salmon fillets skin-side down on a baking sheet and spread 1 tablespoon pesto on each fillet.
4. Roast for 20 minutes.
5. Serve and enjoy!

Nutrition: Per Serving: Net carbs 1 g;Fiber 2 g;Fats 10 g;Fatsr 3 g;Calories 182

Red Snapper Veracruz

Servings:6
Cooking Time: 10 Minutes
Ingredients:
- 10 to 12 multicolored mini bell peppers, stemmed, seeded, and thinly sliced
- 1 (10-ounce) container cherry tomatoes, halved
- 1 cup fresh cilantro, roughly chopped
- 2 tablespoons capers
- Juice of 2 limes
- 2 tablespoons of extra-virgin olive oil
- 1 jalapeño pepper, stem and seeds removed, finely diced
- 4 (4-ounce) snapper fillets
- Post-Op
- 2 to 4 ounces
- 4 ounces

Directions:
1. Preheat a grill to medium-low. Alternatively, preheat the oven to 425°F.
2. In a small mixing bowl, combine the mini bell peppers, tomatoes, cilantro, capers, lime juice, olive oil, and jalapeño pepper to make the salsa. Set aside.
3. Put four large sheets of aluminum foil (about 8½-by-11 inches in size) on a work surface. Place a fish fillet on a foil sheet and top it with one-fourth of the salsa. Fold over the foil so it covers the fish completely, and roll the edges to tightly seal and prevent any air (and liquid) from escaping. Repeat for the remaining three fillets and salsa.
4. Put the foil packets on the grill and close the lid. (The grill temperature should reach no hotter than 450°F.) Cook for 8 to 10 minutes, or until the fish is opaque. The fish is done when it flakes easily with a fork or reaches an internal temperature of 145°F. If using the oven, place the foil packets on a nonstick baking sheet and bake 12 to 15 minutes, or until the fish flakes easily with a fork.

Nutrition: Per Serving (4 ounces): Calories: 161; Total fat: 8g; Protein: 1; Carbs: 7g; Fiber: 1g; Sugar: 4g; Sodium: 137mg

Lime Shrimp

Servings: 2
Cooking Time: 10 Minutes
Ingredients:
- 28 Shrimps, ready to cook
- 1 tablespoon, Lime juice
- 1/8 teaspoon, Salt
- ¾ teaspoon, Black pepper
- 2 tablespoons, Chopped onion
- Cooking spray

Directions:
1. Spray some cooking oil into the skillet.
2. Bring the skillet to medium heat.
3. When the skillet becomes hot, put all the ingredients and sauté occasionally until the onions and shrimps get cooked well.
4. Serve hot

Nutrition:Per Serving: Net carbs 2.2 g;Fiber 0.4 g;Fats 0.9 gSugar 1 g;Calories 84.4

Herb-crusted Salmon

Servings:2
Cooking Time: 20 Minutes
Ingredients:
- 2 (4-ounce) salmon fillets
- 2 teaspoons minced garlic
- 1 tablespoon dried parsley
- ½ teaspoon dried thyme
- 2 teaspoons freshly squeezed lemon
- 4 tablespoons grated Parmigiano-Reggiano cheese
- Post-Op
- 2 ounces
- 4 ounces

Directions:
1. Preheat the oven to 425°F. Line a rimmed baking sheet with parchment paper.
2. Place the salmon skin-side down on the baking sheet and cover with a second piece of parchment paper. Bake for 10 minutes.
3. Meanwhile, mix together the garlic, parsley, thyme, lemon juice, and Parmigiano-Reggiano cheese in a small dish.
4. Discard the parchment paper covering the salmon. Use a pastry brush to carefully cover the fillets with the herb-cheese mixture.
5. Bake the salmon, uncovered, for about 5 minutes more. The salmon is done when the fish flakes easily with a fork.
6. Serve immediately.

Nutrition: Per Serving (4 ounces): Calories: 19 Total fat: 10g; Protein: 27g; Carbs: 9g; Fiber: 1g; Sugar: 3g; Sodium: 222mg

Lemon Garlic Tilapia

Servings: 4
Cooking Time: 30 Minutes
Ingredients:
- 4 fillets, Tilapia
- 1 tablespoon, Olive oil
- 1 tablespoon, Margarine
- 1 tablespoon, Lemon juice
- ¼ teaspoon, Salt
- 1 teaspoon, Garlic salt
- 1 teaspoon, Parsley flakes, dried
- ¼ teaspoon, Cayenne pepperCooking spray

Directions:
1. Set the temperature of the oven at 400°F and start preheating.
2. Spray nonstick cooking oil onto the baking tray.
3. Put the butter into a nonstick saucepan and melt it on low-medium heat.
4. Now, add some lemon juice, salt, olive oil, garlic powder, and parsley into it and sauté for 3-minutes.
5. Place the tilapia fillets in the baking tray and pour the preparation on the top of the fillets.Now sprinkle some cayenne pepper on the fish.
6. Put in the oven and bake for about 12-13 minutes.
7. Flip sides and cook it for extra time.
8. Serve hot

Nutrition:Per Serving: Net carbs 1.8 g;Fiber 0.3 g;Fats 7.3 g;Fatsr 3 g;Calories 175.2

Honey And Soy Glazed Salmon

Servings: 2
Cooking Time: 7 Minutes
Ingredients:
- 2 filets, Salmon
- 2 tablespoons, Honey
- 1½ tablespoons, Lime juice
- 2 tablespoons, Soy sauce, low sodium
- 2 tablespoons, Vegetable oil
- 2 teaspoons, Mustard
- 1 tablespoon, Water

Directions:
1. In a medium bowl, whisk honey, soy sauce, mustard, lime juice, and water.
2. Pour vegetable oil into a non-stick skillet and bring to high heat.
3. Roast the filets at least for 2 to minutes and flip sides and continue roasting for another 2-3 minutes, until it becomes brown.
4. Transfer filets into a serving plate.
5. Add some honey glaze to the skillet and heat for one minute.
6. Pour the honey glaze over salmon and serve hot.

Nutrition:Per Serving: Net carbs 21.3 g;Fiber 0.g;Fats 11.2 g;Fatsr 2 g;Calories 277.3 g

Herb-crusted Salmon Fillets

Servings:4
Cooking Time: 10 Minutes
Ingredients:
- 16 ounces, Atlantic salmon
- 2 tablespoons, Chives, roughly chopped
- 2 tablespoons, Parsley, chopped
- 1 cup, Breadcrumbs, whole-grain
- ½ teaspoon, Garlic powder
- ½ teaspoon, Onion powder
- 1 teaspoon, Lemon peel, grated
- ¼ cup, Lemon juice¼ teaspoon, Salt
- ½ teaspoon, Pepper
- Cooking spray.

Directions:

1. Preheat the oven on high heat at 400°F.
2. Line the baking tray with a baking paper and spray some cooking oil.
3. Season the salmon fillets with pepper and salt.
4. Place the salmon on the baking tray, skin side down facing the baking liner.Put all the ingredients except lemon juice in mixer bowl.
5. Combine well until it becomes a smooth mix.
6. Drizzle some lemon juice on the salmon fillets and spread the breadcrumb mixture over the salmon fillets.
7. Spray evenly with cooking spray, and bake it at least for 10 - 15 minutes.
8. Serve hot.

Nutrition:Per Serving: Net carbs 7.2 g;Fiber 1.1 g;Fats 14.4 g;Fatsr 2 g;Calories 255

Pork Recipes

Pork, White Bean, And Spinach Soup

Servings:4 To 6
Cooking Time: 40 Minutes
Ingredients:
- 1 teaspoon extra-virgin olive oil
- 1 medium onion, chopped
- 2 (4-ounce) boneless pork chops, cut into 1-inch cubes
- 1 (14.5 ounce) can diced tomatoes
- 3 cups low-sodium chicken broth
- ½ teaspoon dried thyme
- ¼ teaspoon crushed red pepper flakes
- 1 (15-ounce) can great northern beans, drained and rinsed
- 8 ounces fresh spinach leaves
- Post-Op
- 1 cup

Directions:
1. Place a large soup pot or Dutch oven over medium heat and heat the olive oil.
2. Add the onion and sauté for 2 to 3 minutes, or until tender. Add the pork and brown it for 4 to 5 minutes on each side.
3. Mix in the tomatoes, broth, thyme, red pepper flakes, and beans. Bring to a boil and then reduce the heat to low to simmer, covered, for 30 minutes.
4. Add the spinach and stir until wilted, about 5 minutes, and serve immediately.
Nutrition: Per Serving (1 cup): Calories: 1; Total fat: 4g; Protein: 17g; Carbs: 17g; Fiber: 4g; Sugar: 6g; Sodium: 600mg

Slow Cooker Pork With Red Peppers And Pineapple

Servings:4
Cooking Time: 5 Hours
Ingredients:
- ¼ cup low-sodium soy sauce or Bragg Liquid Aminos
- Juice of ½ lemon
- 1 teaspoon garlic powder
- 1 teaspoon ground cumin
- ½ teaspoon cayenne pepper
- ¼ teaspoon ground coriander
- 1½ pounds boneless pork tenderloin
- 2 red bell peppers, thinly sliced
- 2 (20-ounce) cans pineapple chunks in 100% natural juice or water, drained
- Post-Op
- 2 to 4 ounces

Directions:
1. In a small bowl, mix together the soy sauce, lemon juice, garlic powder, cumin, cayenne pepper, and coriander.
2. Place the pork tenderloin in the slow cooker and add the red bell pepper slices. Cover with the pineapple chunks and their juices. Pour the soy sauce mixture on top.
3. Cover the slow cooker and turn on low for about 5 hours.
4. Shred the pork with a fork and tongs and continue to cook on low for 20 minutes more, or until juices are absorbed.
5. Serve and enjoy!
Nutrition: Per Serving (3 ounces): Calories: 131; Total fat: 2g; Protein: 17g; Carbs: 11g; Fiber: 2g; Sugar: 8g; Sodium: 431mg

Brown Sugar-mustard Pork Chops

Servings: 6
Cooking Time: 30 Minutes
Ingredients:
- 6 Boneless pork loin chops
- ¼ cup, Yellow mustard
- ½ cup, Brown sugar

Directions:
1. In a medium bowl, mix brown sugar and mustard.
2. Wash and clean the pork.
3. Take glass baking tray and spray some non-stick cooking oil.
4. Place the cleaned pork in the tray.
5. Transfer the mix over the pork chops.
6. Set the temperature of the baking oven at 350°F and bake the pork for 30 minutes.Once ready, serve hot.
Nutrition:Per Serving: Net carbs 12.6 g;Fiber 0.5 g;Fats 6.5 g;Fatsr g;Calories 298

Chipotle Shredded Pork

Servings: 8
Cooking Time: 6 Hours 10 Minutes
Ingredients:
- 1 can chipotle pepper in adobo sauce
- 1 ½ tablespoon apple cider vinegar
- 1 tablespoon ground cumin
- 1 tablespoon dried oregano
- Juice of 1 lime
- 2 pounds pork shoulder, trimmed

Directions:
1. Take your blender and puree chipotle pepper, adobo sauce, apple cider vinegar, cumin, oregano, and lime juice.
2. Transfer pork shoulder in the slow cooker and pour the sauce all over.
3. Cover Slow Cooker and cook for 6 hours on low.
4. Shred the pork using forks and enjoy!
Nutrition:Per Serving: Net carbs g;Fiber 1 g;Fats 11 g;Fatsr 3 g;Calories 260

Balsamic-glazed Pork Tenderloin

Servings: 6
Cooking Time: 25 Minutes
Ingredients:
- 1½ pound, Pork tenderloin
- 3 tablespoons, Brown sugar
- ¼ teaspoon, Salt
- 1/8 teaspoon, Black pepper
- ¼ cup, Balsamic vinegar
- 2 tablespoons, Cooking oil

Directions:
1. Wash and clean pork.
2. Pat dry and season the pork with pepper and salt.
3. Set the oven to 425°F.
4. In a skillet pour cooking oil and roast the pork to brown in medium-low heat.
5. Once all the pork turns brown from all side, remove it.Now add balsamic vinegar and add brown sugar.
6. Stir continuously and let all the brown bits remove from the skillet and becomes a glaze.
7. Now put back the pork into the skillet and allow the glaze to coat evenly on the pork piece.
8. Transfer the entire pork coated with brown sugar and balsamic vinegar into a roasting pan and bake it for about 25 minutes.
9. Spread the glaze over the pork frequently.
10. Serve hot.

Nutrition:Per Serving: Net carbs 4.5 g;Fiber 1 g;Fats 2 g;Fatsr 3 g;Calories 222

Pork Chops With Honey & Garlic

Servings: 6
Cooking Time: 20 Minutes
Ingredients:
- 24 ounces, Pork loin chops, fat removed, cut into 6 pieces.
- 1/8 +¼ cup, Honey
- 3 tablespoons, Soy sauce
- 6 cloves, Garlic, finely chopped

Directions:
1. Combine soy sauce, ¼ cup honey, and garlic in a medium bowl.
2. Marinate the chops in the mixture.

3. Bring grill to medium-high temperature and place chops over it.
4. Cover and cook for 20 minutes.
5. Sprinkle the remaining honey over the chops while grilling.

Nutrition:Per Serving: Net carbs 24.9Fiber 0.2 g;Fats 5.9 g;Fatsr 2 g;Calories 3

One-pan Pork Chops With Apples And Red Onion

Servings:4
Cooking Time: 30 Minutes
Ingredients:
- 2 teaspoons extra-virgin olive oil, divided
- 4 boneless center-cut thin pork chops
- 2 small apples, thinly sliced
- 1 small red onion, thinly sliced
- 1 cup low-sodium chicken broth
- 1 teaspoon Dijon mustard
- 1 teaspoon dried sage
- 1 teaspoon dried thyme
- Post-Op
- ½ to 1 pork chop

Directions:
1. Place a large nonstick frying pan over high heat and add 1 teaspoon of olive oil. When the oil is hot, add the pork chops and reduce the heat to medium. Sear the chops for 3 minutes on one side, flip, and sear the other side for 3 minutes, 6 minutes total. Transfer the chops to a plate and set aside.
2. In the same pan, add the remaining 1 teaspoon of olive oil. Add the apples and onion. Cook for 5 minutes or until tender, stirring frequently to prevent burning.
3. While the apples and onion cook, mix together the broth and Dijon mustard in a small bowl.
4. Add the sage and thyme to the pan and stir to coat the onion and apples. Stir in the broth mixture and return the pork chops to the pan. Cover the pan and simmer for 10 to 15 minutes.
5. Let pork chops rest for 2 minutes before cutting.

Nutrition: Per Serving (1 pork chop): Calories: 234; Total fat: 11g; Protein: 20g; Carbs: 13g; Fiber: 3g; Sugar: 9g; Sodium: 290mg

Sweets and Treats

Chocolate Brownies With Almond Butter

Servings:16 Brownies
Cooking Time: 25 Minutes
Ingredients:
- Nonstick cooking spray
- ½ cup cocoa powder
- 1 tablespoon ground flaxseed
- ½ teaspoon ground instant coffee
- ¼ teaspoon baking soda
- ½ cup almond butter
- ¼ cup melted coconut oil
- 2 large eggs
- 1 teaspoon vanilla extract
- ½ cup agave nectar
- Post-Op
- 1 brownie

Directions:
1. Preheat the oven to 325°F. Coat an 8-by-8-inch glass baking dish with the cooking spray.
2. Place the cocoa powder, flaxseed, instant coffee, baking soda, almond butter, coconut oil, eggs, vanilla, and agave nectar in a high-speed blender or food processor. Blend on medium-high until smooth. Pour the batter into the baking dish.
3. Bake for 25 minutes or until a toothpick inserted in the middle comes out clean. Let cool for 10 minutes before cutting into 16 squares.

Nutrition: Per Serving (1 brownie): Calories: 12 Total fat: 9g; Protein: 3g; Carbs: 11g; Fiber: 2g; Sugar: 9g; Sodium: 49mg

Superfood Dark Chocolates

Servings:18 Chocolates
Cooking Time: 25 Minutes
Ingredients:
- 6 ounces dark chocolate chips (60% cacao or higher, such as Ghirardelli dark chocolate chips)
- ¼ cup pumpkin seeds (pepitas), chopped
- ¼ cup unsweetened shredded coconut
- ¼ cup chopped pecans
- ¼ cup unsweetened dried wild blueberries
- 1 teaspoon sea salt
- Post-Op
- 1 chocolate

Directions:
1. Line 1 or 2 baking sheets with parchment paper.
2. Fill a large pot with water and bring it to a boil. Reduce the heat to a simmer and place a stainless steel heat-proof bowl over the top of the boiling water. Add the chocolate chips and stir until melted and smooth. Alternatively, you can use a double boiler or melt the chocolate in the microwave (use 50 percent power and stir frequently to prevent burning).

3. Use a spoon to drizzle the melted chocolate on the sheet pan in small circles (about ¾ tablespoon of chocolate in circles about 2 inches in diameter).
4. Add the pumpkin seeds, coconut, pecans, and dried blueberries to each chocolate circle. Each should hold about ¾ tablespoon of toppings total. Sprinkle with the sea salt.
5. Let the chocolates harden at room temperature or in the refrigerator. Keep them in an airtight container and eat within 2 weeks to maintain maximum freshness.

Nutrition: Per Serving (1 chocolate): Calories: 102; Total fat: 7g; Protein: 3g; Carbs: 8g; Fiber: 2g; Sugar: ; Sodium: 99mg

No-bake Peanut Butter Protein Bites With Dark Chocolate

Servings:25 Bites
Cooking Time: 20 Minutes
Ingredients:
- 1 cup old-fashioned rolled oats
- 1 cup vanilla protein powder
- ¾ cup smooth natural peanut butter
- 2 tablespoons ground flaxseed
- 1 tablespoon chia seeds
- 1 teaspoon vanilla extract
- ¼ cup dark chocolate chips
- ¾ teaspoon stevia baking blend
- 1 tablespoon water (or more or less to reach desired consistency)
- Post-Op
- 1 to 2 bites

Directions:
1. Mix together the oats, protein powder, peanut butter, flaxseed, chia seeds, vanilla, chocolate chips, stevia, and water in a large mixing bowl.
2. Refrigerate for at least 30 minutes.
3. Roll into 25 balls. Store in an airtight container in the refrigerator.
4. Eat within 1 week or freeze.

Nutrition: Per Serving (2 bites): Calories: 181; Total fat: 10g; Protein: 11g; Carbs: 11g; Fiber: 3g; Sugar: 3g; Sodium: 10g

Easy Peanut Butter Cookies

Servings:15 Cookies
Cooking Time: 15 Minutes
Ingredients:
- Nonstick cooking spray
- 1 cup natural smooth peanut butter
- 1 large egg
- ½ cup stevia baking blend
- ½ teaspoon vanilla extract
- Post-Op
- 1 cookie

Directions:
1. Preheat the oven to 350°F. Coat a nonstick baking sheet with the cooking spray or use parchment paper.
2. In a medium bowl, use a hand mixer to combine the peanut butter, egg, stevia, and vanilla.
3. Roll the batter into 1-inch balls and place them on the baking sheet. Flatten each ball to about ¼-inch thickness. Using a fork, create two imprints of a crisscross pattern on the cookie.
4. Bake for about 12 minutes. The cookies are done when golden brown.
5. Cool for 5 minutes, then move to a baking rack to finish cooling.
Nutrition: Per Serving (1 cookie): Calories: 107; Total fat: 9g; Protein: 4g; Carbs: 4g; Fiber: 1g; Sugar: 2g; Sodium: 47mg

Low-carb Crustless Cherry Cheesecake

Servings:10
Cooking Time: 45 Minutes
Ingredients:
- For the cheesecake
- Nonstick cooking spray
- 2 (8-ounce) packages Neufchâtel cheese, at room temperature
- Juice of ½ lemon
- ¼ cup nonfat plain Greek yogurt
- 2 teaspoons vanilla extract
- ¼ cup stevia baking blend
- 3 large eggs
- For the topping
- 12 ounces frozen cherries, stemmed and pitted
- 2 tablespoons water
- 2 teaspoons cornstarch
- 1 teaspoon stevia baking blend
- Post-Op
- 1 piece (1/10th cheesecake) with cherry topping

Directions:
1. TO MAKE THE CHEESECAKE
2. 1 Preheat the oven to 3°F. Coat a 9-inch springform pan or pie plate with the cooking spray.
3. 2 In a large bowl, mix together the Neufchâtel cheese, lemon juice, yogurt, and vanilla.
4. 3 Add the stevia and mix until smooth.
5. 4 Next mix in the eggs, one at a time, until well blended. Pour the filling into the pan.
6. 5 Bake for 35 to 45 minutes, or until the center is set. When done, the cheesecake should be slightly browned and barely firm in center.
7. TO MAKE THE TOPPING
8. 1 While the cheesecake bakes, place a medium pot over medium-high heat. Put the cherries and water in the pot and bring to a boil, then reduce the heat to medium-low. Simmer until the cherries begin to bubble.
9. 2 Stir 2 tablespoons of the cherry juices into the cornstarch. Stir this slurry into the cherries. This will thicken the topping. Stir in the stevia. Remove the pot from the heat and set aside to cool.
10. 3 Cool the cheesecake for 30 minutes before refrigerating. Refrigerate for at least 2 hours, or overnight, before serving.
11. 4 Serve with the cherry topping.
Nutrition: Per Serving (1 piece with cherry topping): Calories: 156; Total fat: 10g; Protein: 6g; Carbs: 7g; Fiber: 1g; Sugar: 5g; Sodium: 215mg

Old-fashioned Apple Crisp

Servings:10
Cooking Time: 45 Minutes
Ingredients:
- Nonstick cooking spray
- 6 apples, cored, peeled, and cut into 1-inch chunks
- ½ cup water
- 3 teaspoons stevia powder, divided
- 1 tablespoon cornstarch
- ½ teaspoon ground cinnamon
- ¼ teaspoon ground nutmeg
- Juice of ½ lemon
- ¾ cup old-fashioned oats
- ¾ cup whole-wheat pastry flour
- ½ cup low-fat plain Greek yogurt
- ¼ cup coconut oil, melted
- Post-Op
- ½ cup

Directions:
1. Preheat the oven to 350°F. Coat an 8-by-8-inch baking dish with the cooking spray.
2. Put the apples, water, 1½ teaspoons of stevia, cornstarch, cinnamon, nutmeg, and lemon juice in the baking dish. Mix together. Bake for 20 minutes.
3. Meanwhile, in a medium bowl, combine the oats, flour, and the remaining 1½ teaspoons of stevia. Mix in the yogurt and coconut oil. Stir until all the flour is mixed and moistened throughout.
4. Evenly cover the apple mixture with the oatmeal mixture. Bake for 25 minutes more, or until the topping is golden brown.
5. Serve immediately.
Nutrition: Per Serving (½ cup): Calories: 170; Total fat: ; Protein: 3g; Carbs: 28g; Fiber: 5g; Sugar: 8g; Sodium: 7mg

Lemon-blackberry Frozen Yogurt

Servings:4 Cups
Cooking Time: 10 Minutes
Ingredients:

- 4 cups frozen blackberries
- ½ cup low-fat plain Greek yogurt
- Juice of 1 lemon
- 2 teaspoons liquid stevia
- Fresh mint leaves, for garnish
- Post-Op
- ⅔ cup

Directions:
1. In a blender or food processor, add the blackberries, yogurt, lemon juice, and stevia. Blend until smooth, about 5 minutes.
2. Serve immediately or freeze in an airtight container and use within 3 weeks. Garnish with fresh mint leaves.

Nutrition: Per Serving (⅔ cup): Calories: 68; Total fat: 0g; Protein: ; Total Carb: 15g; Fiber: 5g; Sugar: 11g; Sodium: 12mg

Chocolate Chia Pudding

Servings:4
Cooking Time: 15 Minutes
Ingredients:

- 2 cups unsweetened soy milk
- 10 drops liquid stevia
- ¼ cup unsweetened cocoa powder
- ¼ teaspoon ground cinnamon
- ¼ teaspoon vanilla extract
- ½ cup chia seeds
- ½ cup fresh raspberries, for garnish
- Post-Op
- ½ cup

Directions:
1. In a small bowl, whisk together the soy milk, stevia, cocoa powder, cinnamon, and vanilla until well combined.
2. Stir in the chia seeds.
3. Divide between 4 small serving dishes.
4. Cover and refrigerate for at least 1 hour, or overnight.
5. When ready to serve, garnish with the raspberries.

Nutrition: Per Serving (½ cup): Calories 182; Total fat: 9g; Protein: 11g; Carbs: 14g; Fiber: 14g; Sugars: 1g; Sodium: 3g

Dressings, Sauces, and Seasonings

Creamy Peppercorn Ranch Dressing

Servings:1 Cup
Cooking Time: 10 Minutes
Ingredients:
- ¾ cup low-fat plain Greek yogurt
- ⅓ cup grated Parmigiano-Reggiano cheese
- ¼ cup low-fat buttermilk (see here for tip to make from scratch)
- Juice of 1 lemon
- 2 teaspoons freshly ground black pepper
- ½ teaspoon onion flakes
- ¼ teaspoon salt
- Post-Op
- 2 tablespoons

Directions:
1. In a blender or food processor, puree the yogurt, cheese, buttermilk, lemon juice, pepper, onion flakes, and salt on medium-high speed until the dressing is completely smooth and creamy.

Nutrition: Per Serving (tablespoons): Calories: 35; Total fat: 1g; Protein: 4g; Carbs: 2g; Fiber: 0g; Sugar: 1g; Sodium: 133mg

Mango Salsa

Servings:2 Cups
Cooking Time: 15 Minutes
Ingredients:
- 1 large mango, peeled and diced
- ¼ cup fresh cilantro, finely chopped
- Juice of 2 limes
- 1 jalapeño pepper, stemmed, seeded, and diced
- ¼ large red onion, finely diced (about ¼ cup)
- Post-Op
- ¼ cup

Directions:
1. In a medium bowl, mix together the mango, cilantro, lime juice, jalapeño, and onion.
2. Enjoy immediately or refrigerate in an airtight container for up to 3 days.

Nutrition: Per Serving (¼ cup): Calories: 27; Total fat: 0g; Protein: 0g; Carbs: 7g; Fiber: 1g; Sugar: 6g; Sodium: 1mg

Seafood Sauce

Servings:2 Cups
Cooking Time: 10 Minutes
Ingredients:
- 1½ cups catsup (free of high-fructose corn syrup)
- 2 tablespoons grated horseradish
- Juice of 1 lemon
- 1 tablespoon Worcestershire sauce
- 1 teaspoon chili powder
- ¼ teaspoon freshly ground black pepper
- Post-Op
- ¼ cup

Directions:
1. In a small bowl, combine the catsup, horseradish, lemon juice, Worcestershire sauce, chili powder, and pepper. Refrigerate, covered, for at least 30 minutes or overnight to let the flavors meld.
2. Serve with shrimp cocktail, oysters, grilled scallops, or other seafood.

Nutrition: Per Serving (¼ cup): Calories: 56; Total fat: 0g; Protein: 0g; Carbs: 14g; Fiber: 0g; Sugar: 10g; Sodium: 445mg

Homemade Enchilada Sauce

Servings:2 Cups
Cooking Time: 10 Minutes
Ingredients:
- 2 tablespoons extra-virgin olive oil
- ¼ cup chopped onion
- 1 teaspoon minced garlic
- 2 tablespoons whole-wheat pastry flour
- 1 tablespoon chili powder
- ½ teaspoon dried oregano
- ½ teaspoon smoked paprika
- 1 teaspoon ground cumin
- 1 cup low-sodium vegetable or chicken broth
- ½ cup water
- 1 medium tomato, seeded and chopped
- Post-Op
- 2 tablespoons

Directions:
1. Place a small saucepan on the stove over medium heat. Add the oil, onion, and garlic. Sauté for 1 to 2 minutes, or until tender.
2. Add the flour. Continue stirring until the onion and garlic are evenly coated.
3. Mix in the chili powder, oregano, paprika, and cumin. Gradually whisk in the broth and water, whisking constantly to prevent lumps from forming.
4. Add the tomato. Cook for 8 to 10 minutes, stirring frequently, or until mixture has thickened. Use an immersion blender to puree the tomato chunks until smooth. Alternatively, transfer the sauce to a blender and puree until smooth.
5. Serve immediately or refrigerate in an airtight container for up to 1 week. You can also freeze and use at a later date.

Nutrition: Per Serving (2 tablespoons): Calories: 37; Total fat: 0g; Protein: 0g; Carbs: 7g; Fiber: 2g; Sugar: 4g; Sodium: 17mg

Marinara Sauce With Italian Herbs

Servings:3 Cups
Cooking Time: 35 Minutes
Ingredients:

- 1 teaspoon extra-virgin olive oil
- 2 teaspoons minced garlic
- ½ large yellow onion, finely diced
- 1 medium red bell pepper, washed, seeded, and finely diced
- 10 to 12 fresh whole tomatoes, chopped, or 1 (28-ounce) can crushed tomatoes
- 1 teaspoon dried oregano
- ¼ teaspoon red pepper flakes
- 1 teaspoon dried basil
- 2 bay leaves
- Post-Op
- 2 to 4 tablespoons
- 4 tablespoons

Directions:
1. Place a saucepan over medium heat.
2. Heat the olive oil and garlic for 1 minute.
3. Add the onion and red bell pepper. Cook for 1 to 2 minutes, stirring frequently, or until tender.
4. Add the tomatoes, oregano, red pepper flakes, and basil. Gently stir to combine.
5. Add the bay leaves.
6. Cover, reduce the heat to medium-low, and let simmer for 30 minutes.
7. Remove the cover and discard the bay leaves.
8. Use an immersion blender to puree the marinara to your desired consistency. Alternatively, transfer the sauce to a blender and pulse to achieve your preferred consistency.

Nutrition: Per Serving (4 tablespoons): Calories: 37; Total fat: 0g; Protein: 0g; Carbs: 7g; Fiber: 2g; Sugar: 4g; Sodium: 17mg

Perfect Basil Pesto

Servings:5 Tablespoons
Cooking Time: 5 Minutes
Ingredients:

- 1 cup fresh basil leaves
- ¼ cup Parmigiano-Reggiano cheese
- 2½ tablespoons extra-virgin olive oil
- 2 tablespoons pine nuts
- 2 tablespoons water
- Post-Op
- 1 tablespoon

Directions:
1. Place the basil, Parmigiano-Reggiano, olive oil, pine nuts, and water in a food processor or blender. Pulse until smooth.
2. Serve immediately or keep in an airtight container before serving.

Nutrition: Per Serving (1 tablespoon): Calories: 99; Total fat: 10g; Protein: 2g; Carbs: 1g; Fiber: 0g; Sugar: 0g; Sodium: 68mg

Greek Salad Dressing

Servings:1 Cup
Cooking Time: 10 Minutes
Ingredients:

- ⅓ cup extra-virgin olive oil
- Juice of 1 lemon
- 4 teaspoons minced garlic
- 1 tablespoon dried oregano
- 1 teaspoon dried basil
- ½ teaspoon freshly ground black pepper
- ½ teaspoon Dijon mustard
- ½ cup red wine vinegar
- Post-Op
- 2 tablespoons

Directions:
1. In a medium bowl, whisk together the olive oil, lemon juice, garlic, oregano, basil, pepper, and mustard. Alternatively, place these ingredients in a dressing shaker bottle and shake until combined.
2. Whisk in the red wine vinegar until emulsified.
3. Serve immediately. Refrigerate any leftovers in an airtight container. When ready to use, let the dressing sit for 10 to 15 minute at room temperature prior to serving in case the oil has solidified. Give it a whisk or a shake before dressing your salad.

Nutrition: Per Serving (2 tablespoons): Calories: 89; Total fat: 9g; Protein: 0g; Carbs: 1g; Fiber: 0g; Sugar: 0g; Sodium: 3mg

Smoothies Recipes

Mixed Melon Cucumber Coolers

Servings: 2
Cooking Time: 10minutes
Ingredients:
- 2 - cups cubed seedless watermelon
- 1 ½ - cups cubed cantaloupe
- 3 - inch piece of cucumber, peeled and cut into chunks, plus extra slices for garnish
- ½ - ounce fresh lime juice
- Club soda

Directions:
1. Join watermelon, melon, cucumber and lime squeeze in a blender and heartbeat until a thick squeeze structure.
2. Fill two glasses with ice and gap the juice equally among the two glasses.
3. Top each glass with shining water and slide a couple of additional cucumber cuts down within the glass for included flavor. Appreciate!
Nutrition: Calories: 120 Carbs: 28g Fat: 0g Protein: 2g

Raspberry And Fig Hibiscus Cooler

Servings: 2
Cooking Time: 10 Minutes
Ingredients:
- 3 - tablespoons dried hibiscus flowers
- 2 - tablespoons raw honey
- ½ - cup fresh raspberries
- 2 - ripe figs
- 3 - sprigs mint plus extra to garnish
- Lime wedges

Directions:
1. Set the hibiscus blooms in a box and spread with 2cups of bubbling water. Let soak for 5mints. Strain the tea into every other box, eliminating the blooms. Include the nectar and mix till disintegrated.
2. Place the tea in the fridge even as you set up the remainder of the beverage. In another container or a combined drink shaker jumble the raspberries, figs, and mint till all-around beaten and fragrant.
3. Include the cooled tea, mix it nicely, and press the blend to dispose of the mash. Share the tea equally among two glasses. Top it with ice a lime wedge and a sprig of mint.
Nutrition: Calories: 110 Carbs: 20g Fat: 3g Protein: 1g

Non-alcoholic Ginger Mimosa

Servings: 4
Cooking Time: 3minutes
Ingredients:
- ½ - fresh orange juice, chilled
- 1 –tsp maple syrup
- 16 – oz ginger ale
- 4 – pieces, fresh ginger, sliced into 1 inch
- 1 - oranges, sliced
- Ice cubes

Directions:
1. Take a pitcher, include squeezed orange, maple syrup and blend well.
2. Presently include ice blocks and shake well once more.
3. Include soda and mix well.
4. Fill two tall glasses with the readied non-alcoholic ginger mimosa.
5. Top with orange cuts, ginger cuts and serve.
Nutrition: Calories: 150 Carbs: 38g Fat: 0g Protein: 1g

Frozen Peach Bellini Mocktail

Servings: 2
Cooking Time: 5minutes
Ingredients:
- 2 - ripe peaches, peeled and sliced
- 1 - cup sparkling apple juice, plus more for serving
- 2 - teaspoons splenda sugar blend
- 1 - teaspoon lime juice

Directions:
1. Spot cut peaches in the cooler for 60mints.
2. Join peaches, 1 cup shimmering squeezed apple, sugar blend, and lime squeeze in a blender and mix until smooth.
3. Fill 2 glasses and include around 1/2 inch of extra shining squeezed apple.
Nutrition: Calories: 138 Carbs: 31g Fat: 0g Protein: 2g

Raspberry Peach Lemonade

Servings: 8
Cooking Time: 15minutes
Ingredients:
- Raspberry peach puree:
- 4 - fresh peaches, pitted, diced into large chunks
- 1 - cup fresh raspberries
- 1 ¼ - cups water
- Simple syrup:
- ½ - cup granulated sugar
- ½ - cup water
- Lemonade:
- 7 - cups cold water
- 1 ¼ - cups fresh lemon juice
- Ice cubes
- Extra raspberries, for garnish optional
- Extra peach slices, for garnish optional
- Mint sprigs, for garnish optional

Directions:
1. Include diced peaches, raspberries and water to a sustenance processor or blender and procedure until pureed.
2. Spot a strainer over a huge blending bowl and empty the peach raspberry puree into the sifter. Utilize the back of a huge spoon to drive the puree around so the fluid falls through the sifter and seeds/skin remain inside the strainer.
3. Dispose of seeds/skin from the sifter and set blending bowl with fluid in it aside.
4. Include granulated sugar and 1/2 cup water to a little pan and warmth over med heat until sugar disintegrates into the water, blending sometimes. The bubble around 3 minutes until the fluid has turned out to be syrupy. Put aside to cool somewhat.
5. Include 7 cups water, lemon squeeze, and ice blocks to a huge pitcher. Blend to join. Pour in cooled straightforward syrup and peach raspberry fluid. Mix to consolidate once more.
6. Store shrouded in the fridge until prepared to serve. Serve chilled with enhancements, whenever wanted

Nutrition: Calories: 150 carbs: 39g fat: 0g protein: 0g

Healthy Pink Drink Strawberry Refresher

Servings: 1
Cooking Time: 5 Minutes
Ingredients:
- 1 - cup unsweetened strawberry sparkling water like bubbly
- ¼ - cup freeze-dried strawberries
- ½ - cup coconut milk from carton

Directions:
1. Pour solidify dried strawberries in a serving cup at that point pour perrier strawberry shining water over. Mix well and let sit for two or three minutes to soak. Add ice to glass at that point pour coconut milk over. Blend and serve.

Nutrition: Calories 313, Fat 7g Carb 56g Sugar 40g

Sides, Snacks & Desserts Recipes

Choco Peanut Cookies

Servings: 24
Cooking Time: 10 Minutes
Ingredients:
- 1 cup peanut butter
- 1 tsp baking soda
- 2 tsp vanilla
- 1 tbsp butter, melted
- 2 eggs
- 2 tbsp unsweetened cocoa powder
- 2/3 cup erythritol
- 1 1/3 cups almond flour

Directions:
1. Preheat the oven to 350 f.
2. Add all ingredients into the mixing bowl and stir to combine.
3. Make 2-inch balls from mixture and place on greased baking tray and gently press down each ball with fork.
4. Bake in oven for 8-10 minutes.
5. Serve and enjoy.
Nutrition: Calories 110;Fat 9 g;Carbohydrates 9 g;Sugar 1.3 g;Protein 4.g;Cholesterol 15 mg

Quinoa Sesame Brittle

Servings: 10
Cooking Time: 30minutes
Ingredients:
- 1 - cup mixed nuts, chopped
- 1/3 - cup uncooked white quinoa
- 1/3 - cup sesame seeds
- 1/8 - teaspoon sea salt
- ½ - cup maple syrup i used medium amber color
- 4 - tablespoons palm sugar
- 2 - tablespoons coconut oil

Directions:
1. Preheat stove to 5 degrees c (325 f). Line a heating sheet with material paper. Ensure you spread the whole surface and every one of the edges.
2. Consolidate quinoa, blended nuts, sesame seeds, and ocean salt in a major bowl. Blend to join. Put in a safe spot.
3. Consolidate coconut oil, maple syrup, and palm sugar in a little pan. Warm over medium-low heat for 2 to ints. Blend at times until the oil and maple syrup are all around joined. It's ok that the palm sugar isn't totally broken up now.
4. Pour the syrup blend onto the dry fixings. Mix to join and blend all the dry fixings with the fluid.
5. Pour everything onto the focal point of the material lined preparing sheet and spread into an even layer with a spatula. Attempt to get it as even as would be prudent. The weak sheet will venture into a more slender layer as it heats.
6. Prepare for 15mints. Turn the dish (180 degrees) once to guarantee notwithstanding searing. Prepare for another 15 to 20mints. Watch cautiously during the most recent 5 minutes to forestall consuming. The fragile is done when it's turned out to be profound brilliant dark colored in shading.
7. Let cool totally. Break into scaled down pieces with your fingers.
8. Store scraps in a fixed pack or holder at room temperature for a multi week, or in the cooler for as long as a multi month.
Nutrition: Calories: 151 carb: 16. protein: 3g fat: 8.7g sugar: 8.7g

Pickle Roll-ups

Servings:about 40 Mini Roll-ups
Cooking Time: 20 Minutes
Ingredients:
- ¼ pound deli ham (nitrate-free), thinly sliced (about 8 slices)
- 8 ounces Neufchâtel cheese, at room temperature
- 1 teaspoon dried dill
- 1 teaspoon onion powder
- 8 whole kosher dill pickle spears
- Post-Op
- 5 roll-ups (1 entire pickle roll-up)

Directions:
1. Get a large cutting board or clean counter space to assemble your roll-ups.
2. Lay the ham slices on the work surface and carefully spread on the Neufchâtel cheese.
3. Season each lightly with the dill and onion powder.
4. Place an entire pickle on an end of the ham and carefully roll.
5. Slice each pickle roll-up into mini rounds about ½- to 1-inch wide.
6. Skew each with a toothpick for easier serving.
Nutrition: Per Serving (1 roll-up): Calories: 86; Total fat: ; Protein: 4g; Carbs: 4g; Fiber: 0 g; Sugar: 2g; Sodium: 540mg

Fresh Mango Smoothie

Servings: 3
Cooking Time: 10 Minutes
Ingredients:
- 1 medium mango, roughly chopped
- 1 cup coconut milk
- 1 tbsp walnuts, chopped
- 1 tsp vanilla extract, sugar-free
- A handful of ice cubes

Directions:
1. Peel the mango and cut into small chunks. Set aside.
2. Now, combine mango, coconut milk, walnuts, and vanilla extract in a blender and process until well combined and creamy. Transfer to a serving glass and stir in the vanilla extract. Add a few ice cubes and serve immediately.

Nutrition:Per Serving: Net carbs 21.7 g;Fiber 7 g;Fats 21 g;Fatsr 4 g;Calories 271

Broccoli Fritters With Cheddar Cheese

Servings: 4
Cooking Time: 20 Minutes
Ingredients:
- 1 cup cheddar cheese, shredded
- 8 ounces broccoli, chopped, steamed and drained
- 2 large eggs, beaten
- 1 tablespoon avocado oil
- 2 tablespoons oat fiber

Directions:
1. Mix together broccoli with cheddar cheese, eggs and oat fiber in a bowl.
2. Heat avocado oil over medium heat in a nonstick pan and add the broccoli mixture in small chunks.
3. Cook for about 5 minutes on both sides until browned and dish onto a platter to serve.

Nutrition: Calories 178;Total fat 12.6g;Saturated fat 6.8g;Cholesterol 123mg;Sodium 236mg;Total carbohydrate 5.3g;Dietary fiber 2g;Total sugars 1.;Protein 12.1g

Pear-cranberry Pie With Oatmeal Streusel

Servings: 6
Cooking Time: 1 Hr. 30 Minutes
Ingredients:
- Streusel:
- ¾ c. Oats
- 1/3 c. Stevia
- ½ tsp. Cinnamon
- ¼ tsp. Nutmeg
- 1 tbsp. Cubed butter
- Filling:
- 3 c. Cubed pears
- 2 c. Cranberries
- ½ c. Stevia
- 2½ tbsps. Cornstarch

Directions:
1. Set oven to 350 degrees f.

2. Combine all streusel ingredients in a food processor and process into a coarse crumb.
3. Next, combine all filling ingredients in a large bowl and toss to combine.
4. Transfer filling into pie crust, then top with streusel mix.
5. Set to bake until golden brown (about an hour). Cool and serve.

Nutrition: Calories: 280, Fat: 9g, Carbs: 47g, Protein: 1g

Cheesy Radish

Servings: 5
Cooking Time: 1 Hour
Ingredients:
- 16 oz. Monterey jack cheese, shredded
- 2 cups radish
- ½ cup heavy cream
- 1 teaspoon lemon juice
- Salt and white pepper, to taste

Directions:
1. Preheat the oven to 300of and lightly grease a baking sheet.
2. Heat heavy cream in a small saucepan and season with salt and white pepper.
3. Stir in monterey jack cheese and lemon juice.
4. Place the radish on the baking sheet and top with the cheese mixture.
5. Bake for about 4minutes and remove from the oven to serve hot.

Nutrition: Calories 387;Total fat 32g;Saturated fat 20.1g 1;Cholesterol 97mg;Sodium 509mg;Total carbohydrate 2.;Dietary fiber 0.7g;Total sugars 1.3g;Protein 22.8g

Chia Almond Pudding

Servings: 4
Cooking Time: 5 Minutes
Ingredients:
- 2 tbsp almonds, toasted and crushed
- 1/3 cup chia seeds
- ½ tsp vanilla
- 4 tbsp erythritol
- ¼ cup unsweetened cocoa powder
- 2 cups unsweetened almond milk

Directions:
1. Add almond milk, vanilla, sweetener, and cocoa powder into the blender and blend until well combined.
2. Pour blended mixture into the bowl.
3. Add chia seeds and whisk for 1-2 minutes.
4. Pour pudding mixture into the serving bowls and place in fridge for 1-2 hours.
5. Top with crushed almonds and serve.

Nutrition: Calories 170;Fat 12 g;Carbohydrates 12 g;Sugar 1 g;Protein 7 g;Cholesterol 35 mg

Smoked Tofu Quesadillas

Servings: 4
Cooking Time: 25 Minutes
Ingredients:
- 1 lb. Extra firm sliced tofu
- 12 tortillas
- 2 tbsps. Coconut oil
- 6 slices cheddar cheese
- 2 tbsps. Sundried tomatoes
- 1 tbsp. Cilantro
- 5 tbsps. Sour cream

Directions:
1. Lay one tortilla flat and fill with tofu, tomato, cheese and top with oil. Repeat for as many as you need.
2. Bake for 5 minutes and remove from flame.
3. Top with sour cream.
Nutrition: Calories: 136, Fat: 6g, Carbs: 13g, Protein: 10g

Chia Raspberry Pudding

Servings: 2
Cooking Time: 5 Minutes
Ingredients:
- ¼ tsp vanilla
- ¾ cup unsweetened almond milk
- 1 tbsp erythritol
- 2 tbsp proteins collagen peptides
- ¼ cup chia seeds
- ½ cup raspberries, mashed

Directions:
1. Add all ingredients into the bowl and stir until well combined.
2. Place in refrigerator for overnight.
3. Servings chilled and enjoy.
Nutrition: Calories 102;Fat 6 g;Carbohydrates 13 g;Sugar 1.g;Protein 4 g;Cholesterol 0 mg

Lemonade Cupcakes

Servings: 24
Cooking Time: 20minutes
Ingredients:
- 1 15.25 - oz box of white cake mix
- 1 - cup of water
- 1/3 - cup unsweetened applesauce
- 1 - tbsp lemon zest
- 1 ½ - tbsp sugar-free lemonade mix
- 1 to 8 - oz tub of light whipped topping

Directions:
1. Preheat stove to 350. Line 24 biscuit/cupcake cups with paper liners.
2. In a medium-sized blending bowl, consolidate cake blend, water, fruit purée, lemon pizzazz and 1 tbsp of the sans sugar lemonade blend.
3. Spoon hitter equitably into cupcake cups.
4. Prepare until a toothpick embedded into the inside confesses all, about 17mintes. Move cupcakes quickly to a rack to cool.
5. While cupcakes are cooling, make the icing by consolidating the whipped fixing, and staying 1/2 tbsp without sugar lemonade blend.
6. When cupcakes are totally cool, top with icing and serve.
Nutrition: Calories 100 fat 3g carb 16. sugars 11.2g protein 0.8g

Avocado Detox Smoothie

Servings: 2
Cooking Time: 10 Minutes
Ingredients:
- ½ avocado, peeled, roughly chopped
- 1 tbsp powdered stevia1 banana, peeled, chopped
- 1 cup baby spinach, torn
- 1 tbsp goji berries
- 1 tbsp flaxseed, ground
- 1 tsp turmeric, ground

Directions:
1. Peel the avocado and cut in half. Remove the pit and chop one half into small pieces. Wrap the other half in a plastic foil and refrigerate for later.
2. Peel the banana and cut into thin slices. Set aside.
3. Rinse the spinach thoroughly under cold running water using a colander. Chop into small pieces and set aside.
4. Now, combine avocado, banana, spinach, turmeric, flaxseed, and goji berries in a blender. Process until well combined.
5. Transfer to a serving glass and add few ice cubes.
6. Serve immediately.
Nutrition:Per Serving: Net carbs 28.6 g;Fiber 5 g;Fats 11.8 g;Fatsr 4 g;Calories 221

Grilled Avocado In Curry Sauce

Servings: 2
Cooking Time: 30 Minutes
Ingredients:
- 1 large avocado, chopped
- ¼ cup water
- 1 tbsp curry, ground
- 2 tbsp olive oil
- 1 tsp soy sauce
- 1 tsp fresh parsley, finely chopped
- ¼ tsp red pepper flakes¼ tsp sea salt

Directions:
1. Peel the avocado and cut lengthwise in half. Remove the pit and cut the remaining avocado into small chunks. Set aside.
2. Heat up the olive oil in a large saucepan over a medium-high temperature.
3. In a small bowl, combine ground curry, soy sauce, parsley, red pepper and sea salt. Add water and cook for about 5 minutes, stirring occasionally.
4. Add chopped avocado, stir well and cook for 3 more minutes, or until all the liquid evaporates. Turn off the heat and cover. Let it stand for about 15-20 minutes before serving.
Nutrition:Per Serving: Net carbs 10.8 g;Fiber 7.9 g;Fats 34.1 g;Fatsr 4 g;Calories 338

Mix Berry Sorbet

Servings: 1
Cooking Time: 10 Minutes
Ingredients:
- ½ cup raspberries, frozen
- ½ cup blackberries, frozen
- 1 tsp liquid stevia
- 6 tbsp water

Directions:
1. Add all ingredients into the blender and blend until smooth.
2. Pour blended mixture into the container and place in refrigerator until harden.
3. Servings chilled and enjoy.

Nutrition: Calories 63;Fat 0.8 g;Carbohydrates 1g;Sugar 6 g;Protein 1.7 g;Cholesterol 0 mg

Simple Spinach Dip

Servings:12
Cooking Time: 10 Minutes
Ingredients:
- 1 cup plain nonfat Greek yogurt
- 4 ounces Neufchâtel cheese
- ½ cup olive oil-based mayonnaise
- 2 teaspoons minced garlic
- 1½ teaspoons onion powder
- 1 teaspoon smoked paprika
- ¾ teaspoon freshly ground black pepper
- ¼ teaspoon red pepper flakes
- 2 teaspoons Worcestershire sauce
- 1 (8-ounce) can water chestnuts, drained and finely chopped
- ½ cup chopped scallions
- 1 (10-ounce) package frozen chopped spinach, thawed and squeezed of excess moisture
- Post-Op
- ¼ cup

Directions:
1. In a large bowl, use a hand mixer on low speed to mix the yogurt, Neufchâtel cheese, mayonnaise, garlic, onion powder, paprika, black pepper, red pepper flakes, and Worcestershire sauce.
2. Add the water chestnuts, scallions, and spinach and stir by hand until well combined.
3. Cover and refrigerate for at least 2 hours prior to serving, or overnight.
4. Serve with raw vegetables or whole-grain crackers.

Nutrition: Per Serving (¼ cup): Calories: 71; Total fat: 4g; Protein: 3g; Carbs: ; Fiber: 1g; Sugar: 2g; Sodium: 131 mg

Green Tea Smoothie

Servings: 2
Cooking Time: 10 Minutes
Ingredients:
- 3 tbsp green tea powder
- 1 cup grapes, white
- ½ cup kale, finely chopped
- 1 tbsp honey
- ½ tsp fresh mint, ground
- 1 cup water

Directions:

1. Rinse the grapes under cold running water. Drain and remove the pits. Set aside.
2. Place kale in a large colander and wash thoroughly under cold running water. Drain well and finely chop it into small pieces. Set aside.
3. Combine green tea powder with 2 tablespoons of hot water. Soak for 2 minutes. Set aside.
4. Now, combine grapes, kale, honey, mint, and water in a blender and process until well combined. Stir in the water and tea mixture.
5. Refrigerate 30 minutes before serving.
6. Enjoy!

Nutrition: Net carbs 18.3 g Fiber 2.2 g Fats 0.2 g Sugar 1 g Calories

Moist Avocado Brownies

Servings: 9
Cooking Time: 35 Minutes
Ingredients:
- 2 avocados, mashed
- 2 eggs
- 1 tsp baking powder
- 2 tbsp swerve
- 1/3 cup chocolate chips, melted
- 4 tbsp coconut oil, melted
- 2/3 cup unsweetened cocoa powder

Directions:
1. Preheat the oven to 325 f.
2. In a mixing bowl, mix together all dry ingredients.
3. In another bowl, mix together avocado and eggs until well combined.
4. Slowly add dry mixture to the wet along with melted chocolate and coconut oil. Mix well.
5. Pour batter in greased baking pan and bake for 30-3minutes.
6. Slice and serve.

Nutrition: Calories 20Fat 18 g;Carbohydrates 11 g;Sugar 3.6 g;Protein 3.8 g;Cholesterol 38 mg

Skinny Mug Brownies

Servings: 8
Cooking Time: 1minutes
Ingredients:
- 1 - tablespoon cocoa powder, unsweetened
- 2 - packets truvia
- 2 - tablespoons all-purpose flour
- 3 - tablespoons almond milk

Directions:
1. Spot all fixings in a microwave-safe mug. Blend with a fork or little whisk
2. Microwave on high for 60 seconds
3. Appreciate!

Nutrition: Calories: 97 carbs: 9g fat: 2g protein: 1g

Basil Parmesan Tomatoes

Servings: 6
Cooking Time: 30 Minutes
Ingredients:
- ½ teaspoon dried oregano
- 4 roma tomatoes
- Spices: onion powder, garlic powder, sea salt and black pepper
- ½ cup parmesan cheese, shredded
- 12 small fresh basil leaves

Directions:
1. Preheat the oven to 4250f and grease a baking sheet lightly.
2. Mix together dried oregano, onion powder, garlic powder, sea salt and black pepper in a small bowl.
3. Arrange the tomato slices on a baking sheet and sprinkle with the seasoning blend.
4. Top with parmesan cheese and basil leaves and transfer to the oven.
5. Bake for about 20 minutes and remove from the oven to serve.
Nutrition: Calories 49;Total fat 2.2g;Saturated fat 1.4g;Cholesterol 7mg;Sodium 91mg;Total carbohydrate 4.3g;Dietary fiber 1.2g;Total sugars 2.4g;Protein 3.9g

Jicama Fries

Servings: 2
Cooking Time: 20 Minutes
Ingredients:
- 2 tablespoons avocado oil
- 1 jicama, cut into fries
- 1 tablespoon garlic powder
- ½ cup parmesan cheese, grated
- Salt and black pepper, to taste

Directions:
1. Preheat the air fryer to 4000f and grease the fryer basket.
2. Boil jicama fries for about 10 minutes and drain well.
3. Mix jicama fries with garlic powder, salt and black pepper in a bowl.
4. Place in the fryer basket and cook for about 10 minutes.
5. Dish onto a platter and serve warm.
Nutrition: Calories 145;Total fat 7.8g;Saturated fat 4.4g;Cholesterol 20mg;Sodium 2mg;Total carbohydrate 10.4g;Dietary fiber 4g;Total sugars 2.6g;Protein 10.4g

Roasted Spicy Garlic Eggplant Slices

Servings: 4
Cooking Time: 35 Minutes
Ingredients:
- 2 tablespoons olive oil
- 1 eggplant, sliced into rounds
- 1 teaspoon garlic powder
- Salt and red pepper
- ½ teaspoon Italian seasoning

Directions:
1. Preheat the oven to 4000f and line a baking sheet with parchment paper.
2. Arrange the eggplant slices on a baking sheet and drizzle with olive oil.
3. Season with Italian seasoning, garlic powder, salt and red pepper.
4. Transfer to the oven and bake for about 25 minutes.
5. Remove from the oven and serve hot.
Nutrition: Calories 123;Total fat 9.7g;Saturated fat 1.4g;Cholesterol 0mg;Sodium 3mg;Total carbohydrate 10g;Dietary fiber 5.;Total sugars 4.9g;Protein 1.7g

Caprese Snack

Servings: 4
Cooking Time: 5 Minutes
Ingredients:
- 8 oz. Mozzarella, mini cheese balls
- 8 oz. Cherry tomatoes
- 2 tablespoons green pesto
- Salt and black pepper, to taste
- 1 tablespoon garlic powder

Directions:
1. Slice the mozzarella balls and tomatoes in half.
2. Stir in the green pesto and season with garlic powder, salt and pepper to serve.
Nutrition: Calories 407;Total fat .5g;Saturated fat 7.4g;Cholesterol 30mg;Sodium 343mg;Total carbohydrate 6.3g;Dietary fiber 0.9g;Total sugars 2g;Protein 19.4g

Cheesy Low Carb Creamed Spinach

Servings: 8
Cooking Time: 25 Minutes
Ingredients:
- 2 (10 oz) packages frozen chopped spinach, thawed
- 3 tablespoons butter
- 6 ounces cream cheese
- Onion powder, salt and black pepper
- ½ cup parmesan cheese, grated

Directions:
1. Mix together 2 tablespoons of butter with cream cheese, parmesan cheese, salt and black pepper in a bowl.
2. Heat the rest of the butter on medium heat in a small pan and add onion powder.
3. Sauté for about 1 minute and add spinach.
4. Cover and cook on low heat for about 5 minutes.
5. Stir in the cheese mixture and cook for about 3 minutes.
6. Dish into a bowl and serve hot.
Nutrition: Calories 141;Total fat 12.8g;Saturated fat 8g;Cholesterol 3g;Sodium 182mg;Total carbohydrate 3.5g;Dietary fiber 1.6g;Total sugars 0.5g;Protein 4.8g

Macerated Summer Berries With Frozen Yogurt

Servings: 4
Cooking Time: 20 Minutes
Ingredients:
- 1 c. Sliced strawberries
- 1 c. Blueberries
- 1 c. Raspberries
- 1 tbsp. Stevia
- 1 tsp. Orange zest
- 2 tbsps. Orange juice
- 1-pint low fat yogurt

Directions:
1. Add stevia, orange zest, orange juice and berries to a large bowl.
2. Toss to combine. Set to chill for at least hours.
3. Divide yogurt evenly into 4 serving bowls, top evenly with berry mixture and serve.
Nutrition: Calories: 133, Fat: 1g, Carbs: 28., Protein: 1.3g

Frozen Berry Yogurt

Servings: 6
Cooking Time: 5 Minutes
Ingredients:
- 4 cups frozen blackberries
- 1 tsp vanilla
- 1 tbsp fresh lemon juice
- 1 cup full-fat yogurt

Directions:
1. Add all ingredients into the blender and blend until smooth.
2. Pour blended mixture into the container. Cover and place in the refrigerator for hours.
3. Serve and enjoy.
Nutrition: Calories 60 Fat 0.9 g Carbohydrates 11.6 g Sugar 7 g Protein 1.8 g Cholesterol 0 mg

Collard Greens With Burst Cherry Tomatoes

Servings: 4
Cooking Time: 25 Minutes
Ingredients:
- 1-pound collard greens
- 3 strips bacon, cooked and crisped
- ¼ cup cherry tomatoes
- Salt and black pepper, to taste
- 2 tablespoons chicken broth

Directions:
1. Put the collard greens, cherry tomatoes and chicken broth in a pot and stir gently.
2. Cook for about 8 minutes and season with salt and black pepper.
3. Cook for about 2 minutes and stir in the bacon.
4. Cook for about 3 minutes and dish out into a bowl to serve hot.
Nutrition: Calories 110;Total fat 7.6g;Saturated fat 2.3g;Cholesterol 0mg;Sodium 268mg;Total carbohydrate 6.7g;Dietary fiber 3.9g;Total sugars 0.3g;Protein 7g

Tomato, Basil, And Cucumber Salad

Servings:4
Cooking Time: 15 Minutes
Ingredients:
- 1 large cucumber, seeded and sliced
- 4 medium tomatoes, quartered
- 1 medium red onion, thinly sliced
- ½ cup chopped fresh basil
- 3 tablespoons red wine vinegar
- 1 tablespoon extra-virgin olive oil
- ½ teaspoon Dijon mustard
- ½ teaspoon freshly ground black pepper
- Post-Op
- ½ cup serving

Directions:
1. In a medium bowl, mix together the cucumber, tomatoes, red onion, and basil.
2. In a small bowl, whisk together the vinegar, olive oil, mustard, and pepper.
3. Pour the dressing over the vegetables, and gently stir until well combined.
4. Cover and chill for at least 30 minutes prior to serving.
Nutrition: Per Serving (½ cup): Calories: 72; Total fat: 4g; Protein: 1g; Carbs: 8g; Fiber: 1g; Sugar: 4g; Sodium: g

Cheesecake Fat Bombs

Servings: 24
Cooking Time: 10 Minutes
Ingredients:
- 8 oz cream cheese
- 1 ½ tsp vanilla
- 2 tbsp erythritol
- 4 oz coconut oil
- 4 oz heavy cream

Directions:
1. Add all ingredients into the mixing bowl and beat using immersion blender until creamy.
2. Pour batter into the mini cupcake liner and place in refrigerator until set.
3. Serve and enjoy.
Nutrition: Calories 90;Fat 9.8 g;Carbohydrates 1.g;Sugar 0.1 g;Protein 0.8 g;Cholesterol 17 mg

Garlicky Green Beans Stir Fry

Servings: 4
Cooking Time: 25 Minutes
Ingredients:
- 2 tablespoons peanut oil
- 1-pound fresh green beans
- 2 tablespoons garlic, chopped
- Salt and red chili pepper, to taste
- ½ yellow onion, slivered

Directions:
1. Heat peanut oil in a wok over high heat and add garlic and onions.
2. Sauté for about 4 minutes add beans, salt and red chili pepper.
3. Sauté for about minutes and add a little water.
4. Cover with lid and cook on low heat for about 5 minutes.
5. Dish out into a bowl and serve hot.
Nutrition: Calories 107;Total fat 9g;Saturated fat 1.2g;Cholesterol 0mg;Sodium 8mg;Total carbohydrate 10.9g;Dietary fiber 4.3g;Total sugars 2.3g;Protein 2.5g

Baked Zucchini Fries

Servings:6
Cooking Time: 30 Minutes
Ingredients:
- 3 large zucchini
- 2 large eggs
- 1 cup whole-wheat bread crumbs
- ¼ cup shredded Parmigiano-Reggiano cheese
- 1 teaspoon garlic powder
- 1 teaspoon onion powder
- Post-Op
- 4 zucchini fries

Directions:
1. Preheat the oven to 425°F. Line a large rimmed baking sheet with aluminum foil.
2. Halve each zucchini lengthwise and continue slicing each piece into fries about ½ inch in diameter. You will have about 8 strips per zucchini.
3. In a small bowl, crack the eggs and beat lightly.
4. In a medium bowl, combine the bread crumbs, Parmigiano-Reggiano cheese, garlic powder, and onion powder.
5. One by one, dip each zucchini strip into the egg, then roll it in the bread crumb mixture. Place on the prepared baking sheet.
6. Roast for 30 minutes, stirring the fries halfway through. Zucchini fries are done when brown and crispy.
7. Serve immediately.
Nutrition: Per Serving (4 fries): Calories: ; Total fat: 3g; Protein: 5g; Carbs: 10g; Fiber: 1g; Sugar: 3g; Sodium: 179mg

Chocó Protein Balls

Servings: 15
Cooking Time: 10 Minutes
Ingredients:
- 1 tbsp unsweetened cocoa powder
- 1 tsp vanilla
- 3 tbsp pistachios, chopped
- 1/3 cup chia seeds
- 1 cup almond butter
- 1 ½ cup oats

Directions:
1. Line baking tray with parchment paper and set aside.
2. Add all ingredients into the mixing bowl and mix until well combined.
3. Make small balls from mixture and place on a prepared tray and place it in the refrigerator for overnight.
4. Serve and enjoy.
Nutrition: Calories Fat 2.4 g Carbohydrates 6.7 g Sugar 0.2 g Protein 2.1 g Cholesterol 0 mg

Pepper Jack Brussels Sprouts

Servings: 9
Cooking Time: 20 Minutes
Ingredients:
- 2 pounds brussels sprouts, halved and boiled
- 2 tablespoons garlic, minced
- 3 cups pepper jack cheese, shredded
- 2 tablespoons coconut oil
- 1 cup sour cream

Directions:
1. Heat oil in a skillet on medium heat and add garlic.
2. Sauté for about 1 minute and stir in the sour cream and pepper jack cheese.
3. Cook for about 5 minutes on medium low heat and add brussels sprouts.
4. Stir to coat well and cover with the lid.
5. Cook for about minutes and dish out into a bowl to serve.
Nutrition: Calories 274;Total fat 20.7g;Saturated fat 14.1g;Cholesterol 51mg;Sodium 2mg;Total carbohydrate 10.9g;Dietary fiber 3.8g;Total sugars 2.2g;Protein 13.7g

Matcha Ice Cream

Servings: 2
Cooking Time: 5 Minutes
Ingredients:
- ½ tsp vanilla
- 2 tbsp swerve
- 1 tsp matcha powder
- 1 cup heavy whipping cream

Directions:
1. Add all ingredients into the glass jar.
2. Seal jar with lid and shake for 4-5 minutes until mixture double.
3. Place in refrigerator for 4 hours.
4. Servings chilled and enjoy.

Nutrition: Calories 21Fat 22 g;Carbohydrates 3.8 g;Sugar 0.2 g;Protein 1.2 g;Cholesterol 82 mg

Strawberry Frozen Yogurt Squares

Servings: 8
Cooking Time: 8 Hours
Ingredients:
- 1 c. Barley & wheat cereal
- 3 c. Fat-free strawberry yogurt
- 10 oz. Frozen strawberries
- 1 c. Fat- free milk
- 1 c. Whipped topping

Directions:
1. Set a parchment paper on the baking tray.
2. Spread cereal evenly over the bottom of the tray.
3. Add milk, strawberries and yogurt to blender, and process into a smooth mixture.
4. Use yogurt mixture to top cereal, wrap with foil, and place to freeze until firm (about 8 hours).
5. Slightly thaw, slice into squares and serve.

Nutrition: Calories: 188, Fat: 0g, Carbs: 43.4g, Protein: 4.

Zucchini Pizza Boats

Servings: 2
Cooking Time: 45 Minutes
Ingredients:
- 2 medium zucchinis
- ½ c. Tomato sauce
- ½ c. Shredded mozzarella cheese
- 2 tbsps. Parmesan cheese

Directions:
1. Set oven to 350 degrees f.
2. Slice zucchini in half lengthwise and spoon out the core and seeds to form boats.
3. Place zucchini halves skin side down in a small baking dish.
4. Add remaining ingredients inside the hollow center then set to bake until golden brown and fork tender (about 30 minutes).
5. Serve and enjoy.

Nutrition: Calories: 214, Fat: 7.9g, Carbs: 23., Protein: 15.2g

Parmesan Garlic Oven Roasted Mushrooms

Servings: 6
Cooking Time: 30 Minutes
Ingredients:
- 3 tablespoons butter
- 12 oz. Baby bella mushrooms
- ¼ cup pork rinds, finely ground
- Pink Himalayan salt and black pepper, to taste
- ¼ cup parmesan cheese, grated

Directions:
1. Preheat the oven to 4000f and lightly grease a baking sheet.
2. Heat butter in a large skillet over medium high heat and add mushrooms.
3. Sauté for about minutes and dish out.
4. Mix together pork rinds, parmesan cheese, salt and black pepper in a bowl.
5. Put the mushrooms in this mixture and mix to coat well.
6. Place on the baking sheet and transfer to the oven.
7. Bake for about 15 minutes and dish out to immediately serve.

Nutrition: Calories 94;Total fat 7.7g;Saturated fat 4.7g;Cholesterol 22mg;Sodium 22g;Total carbohydrate 3g;Dietary fiber 0.9g;Total sugars 1g;Protein 4.5g

Choco Frosty

Servings: 4
Cooking Time: 5 Minutes
Ingredients:
- 1 tsp vanilla
- 8 drops liquid stevia
- 2 tbsp unsweetened cocoa powder
- 1 tbsp almond butter
- 1 cup heavy cream

Directions:
1. Add all ingredients into the mixing bowl and beat with immersion blender until soft peaks form.
2. Place in refrigerator for 30 minutes.
3. Add frosty mixture into the piping bag and pipe in serving glasses.
4. Serve and enjoy.

Nutrition: Calories 240;Fat 2g;Carbohydrates 4 g;Sugar 3 g;Protein 3 g;Cholesterol 43 mg

Cinnamon Almond Balls

Servings: 12
Cooking Time: 5 Minutes
Ingredients:
- 1 tsp cinnamon
- 3 tbsp erythritol
- 1 ¼ cup almond flour
- 1 cup peanut butter
- Pinch of salt

Directions:
1. Add all ingredients into the mixing bowl and mix well.
2. Cover and place bowl in fridge for 30 minutes.
3. Make small bite size ball from mixture and serve.

Nutrition: Calories 160;Fat 12 g;Carbohydrates 5 g;Sugar 1 g;Protein 6 g;Cholesterol 0 mg

Spicy Tuna Rolls

Servings: 2
Cooking Time: 15 Minutes
Ingredients:
- 1 pouch star-kist selects e.v.o.o. Wild caught yellowfin tuna
- 1 medium cucumber, thinly sliced lengthwise
- 1 teaspoon hot sauce
- 2 slices avocado, diced
- Cayenne, salt and black pepper

Directions:
1. Mix together tuna with hot sauce, cayenne, salt and black pepper in a bowl until combined.
2. Put the tuna mixture on the cucumber slices and top with avocado.
3. Roll up the cucumber and secure with 2 toothpicks to serve.
4. Nutrition Calories 139;Total fat 6.5g;Saturated fat 1.2g;Cholesterol 22mg;Sodium 86mg;Total carbohydrate 8.;Dietary fiber 2.9g;Total sugars 2.8g

Ginger Peach Smoothie

Servings: 4
Cooking Time: 5 Minutes
Ingredients:
- 1 cup coconut milk
- 1 large peach, chopped
- 1 tbsp coconut oil
- 1 tbsp chia seeds
- 1 tsp fresh ginger, peeled

Directions:
1. Wash the peach and cut into half. Remove the pit and chop into bite-sized pieces. Set aside.
2. Cut small ginger knob. Peel it and chop into small pieces. Set aside.
3. Now, combine peach, ginger, coconut milk, and coconut oil in a blender. Process until well combined. Transfer to a serving glass and stir in the chia seeds.
4. Enjoy!

Nutrition:Per Serving: Net carbs 8.9 g;Fiber 3.g;Fats 19 g;Fatsr 6 g;Calories 201

Mixed Berry Popsicles

Servings: 10
Cooking Time: 5 Minutes
Ingredients:
- 1 cup fresh blackberries
- 1 cup fresh blueberries
- 1 cup fresh raspberries
- 2 tbsp fresh lemon juice
- 2 cups strawberries, sliced
- 2 tbsp honey

Directions:
1. Add all ingredients into the blender and blend until smooth.
2. Pour blended mixture into the popsicle molds and place in the freezer for 4 hours or until set.
3. Serve and enjoy.

Nutrition: Calories Fat 0.3 g Carbohydrates 10.7 g Sugar 7.6 g Protein 0.7 g Cholesterol 0 mg

Red Orange Salad

Servings: 3
Cooking Time: 20 Minutes
Ingredients:
- Fresh lettuce leaves, rinsed
- 1 small cucumber sliced
- ½ red bell pepper, sliced
- 1 cup frozen seafood mix
- 1 onion, peeled, finely chopped
- 3 garlic cloves, crushed
- ¼ cup fresh orange juice
- 5 tbsp extra virgin olive oil
- Salt to taste

Directions:
1. Heat up 3 tbsp of extra virgin olive oil over medium-high temperature. Add chopped onion and crushed garlic. Stir fry for about 5 minutes.
2. Reduce the heat to minimum and add 1 cup of frozen seafood mix. Cover and cook for about 15 minutes, until soft. Remove from the heat and allow it to cool for a while.
3. Meanwhile, combine the vegetables in a bowl. Add the remaining 2 tbsp of olive oil, fresh orange juice and a little salt. Toss well to combine.
4. Top with seafood mix and serve immediately.

Nutrition:Per Serving: Net carbs 13.1 g;Fiber 1.8 g;Fats 14.6 g;Fatsr 4 g;Calories 206

Italian Eggplant Pizzas

Servings:6
Cooking Time: 30 Minutes
Ingredients:
- 1 large eggplant, cut into ¼- to ½-inch rounds
- 1 tablespoon salt
- 1 tablespoon extra-virgin olive oil
- 2 teaspoons minced garlic
- ½ teaspoon dried oregano
- 1 cup Marinara Sauce with Italian Herbs
- 1 cup fresh basil leaves
- 1 cup shredded part-skim Mozzarella cheese
- ¼ cup shredded Parmigiano-Reggiano cheese
- Post-Op
- 1 to 2 eggplant pizza rounds
- 2 to 4 eggplant pizza rounds

Directions:
1. Preheat the oven to 425°F. Line a large rimmed baking sheet with aluminum foil.
2. Put the eggplant rounds on paper towels and sprinkle them with the salt. Let them sit for 10 to 15 minutes to help release some of the water in the eggplant. Pat dry afterward. It's okay to wipe off some of the salt before baking.
3. In a small bowl, mix together the olive oil, garlic, and oregano.
4. Place the eggplant rounds 1-inch apart on the baking sheet. Using a pastry brush, coat each side of the eggplant with the olive oil mixture. Bake the eggplant for 15 minutes.
5. Create pizzas by layering 1 to 2 tablespoons of marinara sauce, 2 basil leaves, about 1 tablespoon of mozzarella cheese, and about ½ tablespoon of Parmigiano-Reggiano cheese on each baked eggplant round.
6. Bake the pizzas for an additional 10 minutes or until the cheese is melted and starting to brown.
7. Serve immediately and enjoy!

Nutrition: Per Serving (2 eggplant pizza rounds): Calories: 99; Total fat: 6g; Protein: 5g; Carbs: 7g; Fiber: 2g; Sugar: 4g; Sodium: 500mg

Raspberry Sorbet

Servings: 4
Cooking Time: 5 Minutes
Ingredients:
- 12 oz frozen raspberries
- 1 tbsp honey
- ¼ cup of coconut water

Directions:
1. Add all ingredients into the blender and blend until smooth.
2. Pour blended mixture into the container. Cover and place in the freezer for 3 hours.
3. Serve and enjoy.

Nutrition: Calories 61 Fat 0.1 g Carbohydrates 15.5 g Sugar 13.3 g Protein 0.g Cholesterol 0mg

Crispy Baked Zucchini Fries

Servings: 4

Cooking Time: 30 Minutes
Ingredients:
- ¾ cup parmesan cheese, grated
- 2 medium zucchinis, chopped into small ticks
- 1 large egg
- ¼ teaspoon black pepper
- ¼ teaspoon garlic powder

Directions:
1. Preheat the oven to 4250f and grease a baking sheet lightly.
2. Whisk egg in one bowl and mix together parmesan cheese, black pepper and garlic powder in another bowl.
3. Dip each zucchini stick in the egg and then dredge in the dry mixture.
4. Transfer to the baking sheet and place in the oven.
5. Bake for about 20 minutes until golden and broil for 3 minutes to serve.

Nutrition: Calories 102;Total fat 5.9g;Saturated fat 3.4g;Cholesterol mg;Sodium 222mg;Total carbohydrate 4.3g;Dietary fiber 1.1g;Total sugars 1.8g;Protein 9.6g

Broccoli Cauliflower Puree

Servings: 2
Cooking Time: 20 Minutes
Ingredients:
- 2 cups fresh broccoli chopped
- 2 cups fresh cauliflower, chopped
- ½ cup skim milk½ tsp salt
- ½ tsp Italian seasoning
- ¼ tsp cumin, ground
- 1 tbsp fresh parsley, finely chopped
- 1 tbsp olive oil
- 1 tsp dry mint, ground

Directions:
1. Wash and roughly chop the cauliflower. Place it in a deep pot and add a pinch of salt. Cook for about -20 minutes. When done, drain and transfer it to a food processor. Set aside.
2. Wash the broccoli and chop into bite-sized pieces. Add it to the food processor along with milk, salt, Italian seasoning, cumin, parsley, and mint. Gradually add olive oil and blend until nicely pureed.
3. Serve with some fresh carrots and celery.

Nutrition: Per Serving: Net carbs 12.7 g;Fiber 6 g;Fats 7.5 g;Fatsr 2 g;Calories 138

Avocado Hummus

Servings: 4
Cooking Time: 5 Minutes
Ingredients:
- ½ avocado, chopped
- 2 tbsp olive oil
- ½ tsp onion powder
- 1 tsp tahini
- ½ tsp garlic, minced
- 1 tbsp lemon juice
- 1 cup frozen edamame, thawed
- Pepper
- Salt

Directions:
1. Add all ingredients into the blender and blend until smooth.
2. Serve with vegetables.

Nutrition: Calories 215 Fat 17 g Carbohydrates 10 g Sugar 0.g Protein 9.1 g Cholesterol 0 mg

Chocolate Ice Cream

Servings: 8
Cooking Time: 30 Minutes
Ingredients:
- 4 4oz vanilla and chocolate yogurt
- 2/3 cup low-fat custard
- 2 tbsp. low-fat hot chocolate powder
- 2 scoops flavorless protein powder
- 2/3 cup skim milk

Directions:
1. Mix the yogurt, chocolate powder, protein powder, milk, and custard together.
2. Pour the mixture into a freezer safe bowl and allow it to freeze until it has completely firmed up. Whisk the mixture every 30 minutes. This will ensure that large ice crystals don't form and it has more of an ice cream consistency. If you have an ice cream maker, you can place the mixture into it and mix before you place it in the freezer.
3. Before you serve, you should let it set for around minutes to soften just a bit.

Nutrition:Per Servings: Calories: 352, Sodium: 111mg, Cholesterol: 161mg, Protein: , Carbohydrates: 26.9g, Fat: 26.7g

Beet Spinach Salad

Servings: 3
Cooking Time: 40 Minutes
Ingredients:
- 2 medium-sized beet, trimmed, sliced
- 1 cup fresh spinach, chopped
- 2 spring onions, finely chopped
- 1 small green apple, cored, chopped
- 3 tbsp olive oil
- 2 tbsp fresh lime juice
- 1 tbsp honey, raw
- 1 tsp apple cider vinegar
- 1 tsp salt

Directions:
1. Wash the beets and trim off the green parts. Set aside.
2. Wash the spinach thoroughly and drain. Cut into small pieces and set aside.
3. Wash the apple and cut lengthwise in half. Remove the core and cut into bite-sized pieces and set aside.
4. Wash the onions and cut into small pieces. Set aside.
5. In a small bowl, combine olive oil, lime juice, honey, vinegar, and salt. Stir until well incorporated and set aside to allow flavors to meld.
6. Place the beets in a deep pot. Pour enough water to cover and cook for about 40 minutes, or until tender. Remove the skin and slice. Set aside.
7. In a large salad bowl, combine beets, spinach, spring onions, and apple. Stir well until combined and drizzle with previously prepared dressing. Give it a good final stir and serve immediately.

Nutrition:Per Serving: Net carbs 23.g;Fiber 3.6 g;Fats 14.3 g;Fatsr 5 g;Calories 215

Pumpkin Pie Spiced Yogurt

Servings: 2
Cooking Time: 15 Minutes
Ingredients:
- 2 cup low fat plain yogurt
- ½ cup pumpkin puree
- ¼ tsp. Cinnamon
- ¼ tsp. Pumpkin pie spice
- ¼ cup chopped walnuts
- 1 tbsp. Honey

Directions:
1. Combine spices with the pumpkin puree in a medium bowl and stir.
2. Stir in yogurt, divide into serving glasses. Top with honey and walnuts. Serve and enjoy!

Nutrition: Net carbs 22 g Fiber 1 g Fats 7 g Sugar 10 g Calories 208

Chia Seed Pudding

Servings: 4
Cooking Time: 5 Minutes
Ingredients:
- ½ cup chia seeds
- 1 tsp liquid stevia
- 1 ½ tsp pumpkin pie spice
- ½ cup pumpkin puree
- ¾ cup unsweetened coconut milk
- ¾ cup full-fat coconut milk

Directions:
1. Add all ingredients into the mixing bowl and whisk well to combine.
2. Pour into the serving bowls and place them in the refrigerator for hours.
3. Serve and enjoy.

Nutrition: Calories 275 Fat 25 g Carbohydrates 9.9 g Sugar 3.3 g Protein 5.3 g Cholesterol 0 mg

Cherry Chocolate Chip Ice Cream

Servings: 8
Cooking Time: 10minutes
Ingredients:
- 2 - cups cherries, fresh
- ½ - banana
- ½ - cup unsweetened almond milk
- 3 - tablespoons dairy-free chocolate chips

Directions:
1. Spot all fixings in a microwave-secure mug. Blend with a fork
2. Microwave on high for 60seconds
3. Appreciate!
4. Wash and dry the fruits, and take everything out of the pits. Spot in a cooler percent or glass holder, and stop for at any price three hours. In the occasion which you do not have an opportunity, you may make use of solidified end result.
5. Strip a banana, and notice half in the cooler.
6. Pour ¼ cup of the almond milk into ice 3-d rectangular plate, and forestall those additionally, for in any occasion three hours.
7. Spot the solidified end result, a massive part of a solidified banana, the almond-milk ice 3 - d shapes, and ¼ cup almond milk in a nourishment processor, and manner till definitely easy, a few minutes.
8. Blend in chocolate chips, and recognize right away!

Nutrition: Calories: 128, carb: 22.3g, protein: 2.1g, fat: 4, sugar: 17g,

Low Carb Onion Rings

Servings: 6
Cooking Time: 30 Minutes
Ingredients:
- 2 medium white onions, sliced into ½ inch thick rings
- ½ cup coconut flour
- 4 large eggs
- 4 oz pork rinds
- 1 cup parmesan cheese, grated

Directions:
1. Preheat an air fryer to 3900f and grease a fryer basket.
2. Put coconut flour in one bowl, eggs in the second bowl and pork rinds and parmesan cheese in the third bowl.
3. Coat the onion rings through the three bowls one by one and repeat.
4. Place the coated onion rings in the fryer basket and cook for about 15 minutes.
5. Dish out to a platter and serve with your favorite low carb sauce.

Nutrition: Calories 270;Total fat 15.1g;Saturated fat 7.1g;Cholesterol 1mg;Sodium 586mg;Total carbohydrate 11g;Dietary fiber 4.8g;Total sugars 1.8g;Protein 24.1g

Almond Flour Crackers

Servings: 6
Cooking Time: 25 Minutes
Ingredients:
- 2 tablespoons sunflower seeds
- 1 cup almond flour
- ¾ teaspoon sea salt
- 1 tablespoon whole psyllium husks
- 1 tablespoon coconut oil

Directions:
1. Preheat the oven to 3500f and grease baking sheet lightly.
2. Mix together sunflower seeds, almond flour, sea salt, coconut oil, psyllium husks and tablespoons of water in a bowl.
3. Transfer into a blender and blend until smooth.
4. form a dough out of this mixture and roll it on the parchment paper until 1/16 inch thick.
5. slice into 1-inch squares and season with some sea salt.
6. arrange the squares on the baking sheet and transfer to the oven.
7. bake for about 15 minutes until edges are crisp and brown.
8. allow to cool and separate into squares to serve.

Nutrition: Calories 141;Total fat 11.6g;Saturated fat 2.7g;Cholesterol 0mg;Sodium 241mg;Total carbohydrate 5.2g;Dietary fiber 3.1g;Total sugars 0g;Protein 4.2g

Roasted Root Vegetables

Servings:about 6 Cups
Cooking Time: 45 Minutes
Ingredients:
- Nonstick cooking spray
- 2 medium red beets, peeled
- 2 large parsnips, peeled
- 2 large carrots, peeled
- 1 medium butternut squash (about 2 pounds), peeled and seeded
- 1 medium red onion
- 2 tablespoons extra-virgin olive oil
- 4 teaspoons minced garlic
- 2 teaspoons dried thyme
- Post-Op
- ¼ cup serving
- ½ to 1 cup serving

Directions:
1. Preheat the oven to 425°F. Spray a large rimmed baking sheet with the cooking spray.
2. Roughly chop the beets, parsnips, carrots, and butternut squash into 1-inch pieces. Cut the onion into half and then each half into 4 large chunks.
3. Arrange the vegetables in a single, even layer on the baking sheet, and sprinkle them with the olive oil, garlic, and thyme. Use a spoon to mix the vegetables to coat them with the oil and seasonings.
4. Roast for 45 minutes, stirring the vegetables every 15 minutes, until all the vegetables are tender.
5. Serve immediately.

Nutrition: Per Serving (½ cup): Calories: ; Total fat: 3g; Protein: 1g; Carbs: 11g; Fiber: 1g; Sugar: 5g; Sodium: 30mg

Chocolate Avocado Pudding

Servings: 6
Cooking Time: 10 Minutes
Ingredients:
- 2 avocados, chopped
- ¼ cup creamy almond butter
- 1 tsp vanilla
- 1 tbsp unsweetened cocoa powder
- 1 cup semi-sweet chocolate chips
- 1 cup unsweetened almond milk

Directions:
1. Add chocolate chips and almond milk in a microwave-safe bowl and microwave for 30 seconds. Stir well and microwave for 30 seconds more or until chocolate is melted.
2. Add vanilla and cocoa powder and stir well.
3. Pour chocolate mixture into the blender. Add remaining ingredients and blend until smooth.
4. Pour pudding into the serving bowls and place in the refrigerator for 30 minutes.
5. Serve and enjoy.

Nutrition: Calories 248 Fat 13.4 g Carbohydrates 28.7 g Sugar 21.5 g Protein 3.5 g Cholesterol 0 mg

Cream Cheese Frosting

Servings: 3
Cooking Time: 10 Minutes
Ingredients:
- ½ - cup cream cheese, such as homemade cashew cream cheese
- ½ - tsp pure vanilla extract
- 4 - tbsp powdered sugar
- ¼ - cup silken tofu
- 2 - tbsp milk of choice, as needed for desired thickness

Directions:
1. Mix everything together in a little nourishment processor.
2. In case you're utilizing this formula to top cupcakes, i'd prescribe icing them just before serving, or icing prior and afterward putting away the cupcakes in the refrigerator, because of the short-lived nature of the fixings.
3. Extra icing can be put away for a couple of days in the cooler, secured.
4. Variety thoughts: add pumpkin, or destroyed carrot and pineapple for a carrot cake plunge, or cinnamon and pecans.

Nutrition: Calories: 20, fat: 1., carb: 0.5g protein: 0.5g sugar: 0g

Sweet Pumpkin Pudding

Servings: 4
Cooking Time: 15 Minutes
Ingredients:
- 1 lb. pumpkin, peeled and chopped into bite-sized pieces
- 2 tbsp honey
- ½ cup cornstarch
- 4 cups pumpkin juice, unsweetened
- 1 tsp cinnamon, ground
- 3 cloves, freshly ground

Directions:
1. Peel and prepare the pumpkin. Scrape out seeds and chop into bite-sized pieces. Set aside.
2. In a small bowl, combine pumpkin juice, honey, orange juice, cinnamon, and cornstarch.
3. Place the pumpkin chops in a large pot and pour the pumpkin juice mixture. Stir well and then finally add cloves. Stir until well incorporated and heat up until almost boiling. Reduce the heat to low and cook for about 15 minutes, or until the mixture thickens.
4. Remove from the heat and transfer to the bowls immediately. Set aside to cool completely and then refrigerate for 15 minutes before serving, or simply chill overnight.

Nutrition: Per Serving: Net carbs g; Fiber 4.6 g; Fats 0.9 g; Fatsr 6 g; Calories 232

14-Day Meal Plan

Day 1
Breakfast: Breakfast Kale Muffins
Lunch: Grilled Fig And Peach Arugula Salad With Ricotta Salata And A Black Pepper Vinagretteprint
Dinner: Yummy Chicken Bites

Day 2
Breakfast: Low Carb Cottage Cheese Pancakes
Lunch: Shrimp Scampi
Dinner: Salmon Patties

Day 3
Breakfast: Sweet Millet Congee
Lunch: Stuff Cheese Pork Chops
Dinner: Taco Omelet

Day 4
Breakfast: Vanilla Egg Custard
Lunch: Sheet Pan Spicy Tofu And Green Beans
Dinner: Skillet Chicken Thighs With Potato, Apple, And Spinach

Day 5
Breakfast: Strawberry & Mushroom Sandwich
Lunch: Apple Cider Glazed Chicken Breast With Carrots
Dinner: Onion Paprika Pork Tenderloin

Day 6
Breakfast: Mushroom Frittata
Lunch: Skinny Chicken Pesto Bake
Dinner: Avocado Shrimp Salad

Day 7
Breakfast: Apple And Goat Cheese Sandwich
Lunch: Cheesy Broccoli Soup
Dinner: Creamy Salmon Salad

Day 8
Breakfast: Blueberry Greek Yogurt Pancakes
Lunch: Thyme Oregano Pork Roast
Dinner: Honey & Soy Glazed Radishes

Day 9
Breakfast: Egg White Oatmeal With Strawberries And Peanut Butter
Lunch: Rosemary Garlic Pork Roast
Dinner: Mayo-less Tuna Salad

Day 10
Breakfast: Blackberry Vanilla French Toast
Lunch: Pesto & Mozzarella Stuffed Portobello Mushroom Caps
Dinner: Carrot Sweet Potato Soup

Day 11
Breakfast: Almond Peanut Butter Oatmeal
Lunch: Baked Salmon
Dinner: Creamy Cauliflower Soup

Day 12
Breakfast: Strawberry & Mushroom Breakfast Sandwich
Lunch: Baked Lemon Tilapia
Dinner: Grilled Veal Steak With Vegetables

Day 13
Breakfast: Steel Cut Oat Blueberry Pancakes
Lunch: Coconut Flour Spinach Casserole
Dinner: Baked Cod Cups

Day 14
Breakfast: Berry Cheesecake Overnight Oats
Lunch: Stir-fried Chicken With Corn And Millet
Dinner: Avocado Eggs With Dried Rosemary

Appendix : Recipes Index

Veggie Quesadillas With Cilantro Yogurt Dip 46
Veggie Quiche Muffins 27
Very Berry Muesli 25

W

Watermelon Quinoa Parfait 20
Whole Herbed Roasted Chicken In The Slow Cooker 63
Wild Salmon Salad 80

Wisconsin Scrambler With Aged Cheddar Cheese 17

Y

Yummy Chicken Bites 29

Z

Zoodles With Pesto 51
Zoodles With Turkey Meatballs 62
Zucchini Frittata 29
Zucchini Pizza Boats 100